The Creative Cognitive
Therapy Method

of related interest

Creative Counselling
Creative Tools and Interventions to Nurture Therapeutic Relationships
Tanja Sharpe
Foreword by Suzanne Alderson
ISBN 978 1 83997 018 4
eISBN 978 1 83997 017 7

Creative Approaches to CBT
Art Activities for Every Stage of the CBT Process
Patricia Sherwood
ISBN 978 1 78592 508 5
eISBN 978 1 78450 891 3

The CBT Art Activity Book
100 illustrated handouts for creative therapeutic work
Jennifer Guest
ISBN 978 1 84905 665 6
eISBN 978 1 78450 168 6

THE CREATIVE COGNITIVE THERAPY METHOD

Combining Traditional CBT with Art Therapy for Real Change

Developed and written by
PAMELA HAYES MALKOFF

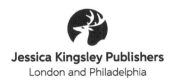

Jessica Kingsley Publishers
London and Philadelphia

First published in Great Britain in 2025 by Jessica Kingsley Publishers
An imprint of John Murray Press

2

Copyright © Pamela Hayes Malkoff 2025

The right of Pamela Hayes Malkoff to be identified as the Author of the Work has been asserted by her in accordance with the Copyright, Designs and Patents Act 1988.

Front cover image source: Nicola Powling. The cover image is for illustrative purposes only, and any person featuring is a model.

A CIP catalogue record for this title is available from the British Library and the Library of Congress

ISBN 978 1 80501 159 0
eISBN 978 1 80501 160 6

Printed and bound in the United States by Integrated Books International

Jessica Kingsley Publishers' policy is to use papers that are natural, renewable and recyclable products and made from wood grown in sustainable forests. The logging and manufacturing processes are expected to conform to the environmental regulations of the country of origin.

Jessica Kingsley Publishers
Carmelite House
50 Victoria Embankment
London EC4Y 0DZ

www.jkp.com

John Murray Press
Part of Hodder & Stoughton Ltd
An Hachette Company

Contents

Acknowledgments

To my editor and dearest friend of almost 30 years, Kelley McKenna. Completing this book has been a journey, and I am immensely grateful to have had you by my side every step of the way. Your unwavering support, keen editorial eye, and friendship have made all the difference. I want to express my deepest gratitude for your dedication to this project. You didn't just edit; you invested your time, expertise, and encouragement. Your insights and candid feedback challenged me to improve and refine the narrative, and I appreciate your honesty throughout this process. Choosing you as my editor was one of the best decisions I made, and I feel truly blessed to have you as both a guide and a friend. This journey has not only resulted in a completed book but also strengthened our friendship in ways I cherish deeply. Thank you, Kelley, for being an indispensable part of this endeavor.

To my wonderful family, a heartfelt gratitude extends to my brother, David, my sister, Amy, and my sister-in-law, Nathalie. Your support and patience as I rambled on about this project did not go unnoticed. If there were moments when you might have grown tired of hearing about it, you graciously kept it to yourselves. Your understanding and encouragement have meant the world to me.

To my beautiful daughters, Sawyer and Cydney, your wisdom and words of encouragement have been my guiding light. Your love inspires me to strive for a better version of myself. Your strength and ability to say just the right thing at precisely the right moment has been a source of comfort and motivation. As I reflect on the love and support within our family, tears of gratitude fill my eyes. Thank you both for embracing this project with open hearts.

To my husband, Greg, your belief in me has been my anchor throughout the journey of creating this book. Your willingness to make time for me, especially when it came to the meticulous tasks of scanning and uploading images, made a world of difference. I am profoundly grateful for your endless support, understanding, and the patience you displayed when I had to prioritize writing over our cherished time together. Thank you for the countless meals you prepared, sustaining me during long writing sessions, and for your gentle reminders to step away from my computer and embrace the beauty of nature. Your encouragement to take breaks, breathe in fresh air, and experience the world beyond the pages has been invaluable.

Introduction

WELCOME TO THE CREATIVE COGNITIVE THERAPY METHOD!

As a therapist, I was frustrated watching my clients not achieving the transformation they desired, but instead getting lost in the minutiae of day-to-day life and losing track of the bigger picture. Therapy is only helpful if approached with an organized, intentional strategy. Otherwise, you're just spending money and time to vent, not to heal. This inspired me to create a program to help both therapists and clients stay focused on the bigger underlying issues. That is how the Creative Cognitive Therapy Method came to be.

Using this workbook as a guide for self-improvement

I want to acknowledge how proud I am of you for showing up and making a commitment to your mental health. I have over 30 years' experience and I know, without a shadow of a doubt, that you can get to a place where you feel much better. If you've picked up this workbook for yourself, rest assured that the *Creative Cognitive Therapy Method Workbook* is specifically designed for independent progression through each step of your journey. To maximize your progress, it's crucial to methodically work through all the modules in the prescribed order. Allocate sufficient time for completing the exercises, and for journaling, which will help you to effectively process your experiences. Remember that each module builds upon the previous one, so it's essential not to skip any sections.

If you've purchased this workbook as a therapist aiming to utilize the Creative Cognitive Therapy Method (CCTM) with your clients, you'll find valuable guidance at the end of each chapter on how to effectively incorporate this material into your therapy sessions. The Creative Cognitive Therapy Method is an intentional and strategic system that combines two psychological methods of equal value and complementary foundations: Cognitive Behavioral Therapy (CBT) and Art Therapy.

Cognitive Behavioral Therapy is an evidence-based practice, which research has shown to be effective in treating a variety of issues such as anxiety, depression, and PTSD.[1] By learning how to identify and challenge negative thought patterns, you can begin to make positive changes in your life. CBT addresses distortions in thinking, which are also known as cognitive distortions. These distortions can lead to negative emotions and behaviors and can ultimately impact an individual's overall well-being. CBT works to identify the negative thoughts that arise in certain situations and examines the evidence that supports or contradicts those thoughts. A person can then develop alternative, more balanced thoughts that are grounded in reality.

However, like any approach to therapy, there are some potential downsides to consider with CBT. Some people think that it is too focused on the individual's thoughts and behaviors and neglects the importance of emotions. This is where Art Therapy combined with CBT can work wonders!

One of the primary benefits of Art Therapy is its ability to facilitate emotional expression and insight. Art (paint, clay, markers, etc.) provides a means of communicating feelings that may be difficult to articulate with words alone. Through the use of colors, lines, shapes, and composition, clients are able to externalize their inner thoughts and feelings in a safe and non-threatening manner. This process allows for deeper understanding of the self and can lead to increased awareness and personal growth. Art

Therapy also provides a space for you to explore your creativity and experiment with alternate ways of problem-solving because making art can stimulate the brain in new ways, allowing for the creation of fresh neural connections and the development of multiple perspectives. Through this process, you may gain new insights that lead to creative solutions for addressing challenges in your life.

Some people may ask: What if I'm not an artist? Yes, making art can be intimidating! You may fear not being "good enough" at something you've never done before. This could create a barrier and make it hard to begin. However, it's essential to note that the focus of Art Therapy is not the final product, but the process of creation itself. In Art Therapy, there is no "right" or "wrong" way to make art. Art-making is especially beneficial for individuals who find it difficult to express themselves verbally. The creative process can foster a sense of accomplishment and enhance self-esteem as individuals witness their works of art come to fruition. Art Therapy offers a visual representation of thoughts and emotions, providing a unique outlet for self-expression and growth. It offers a non-judgmental environment where imperfection is welcomed. The focus is not on the aesthetic qualities of the artwork but on the emotional experience and feelings elicited during the creative process. Even when the outcome appears unpleasing, it presents an opportunity for individuals to confront frustration and learn to persist despite challenges. In this safe space, the emphasis is on self-expression and personal growth, rather than external validation.

In my 30+ years as a Board-Certified Art Therapist I have often been asked: "Why should I make art?" My answer has changed over the years, but I have come to believe there are five basic benefits, and here they are:

- *Artistic creation offers a form of cognitive stimulation, challenging your brain in new and unique ways.* By engaging in activities that are outside your usual routine, you foster the development of new neural connections, which can result in increased flexibility when facing problems or making decisions. As a result, you may be better equipped to identify multiple perspectives and options, having exercised your brain's problem-solving abilities through the art-making process.[2]

- *Art offers a respite from the complexities of daily life by demanding one's full attention.* Whether you're engaging in drawing, painting, sculpting, or collaging, the art-making process requires focus and concentration, making it impossible for your brain to focus on other worries. This can provide a release from anxiety, pain, and stress as you become fully immersed in the moment. Art-making is a mindful activity that helps to quiet the inner thoughts that contribute to anxiety and promotes presence in the now.

- *Art can serve as a means of expressing innermost feelings, fears, and fantasies.* Though exploring one's subconscious can be intimidating, drawing or painting those internal thoughts can provide an alternative way of telling your story. Through this creative process, you may uncover new insights about yourself and gain a deeper understanding of your emotions. Sometimes, art can even lead to a transformative "a-ha" moment.

For instance, one of my clients, Susan, sought therapy because she had been feeling unwell and had a persistent sense that something was wrong, yet she couldn't pinpoint the source of her unease. She described feeling constantly tired and lacking motivation, which we initially both assumed was depression. In an attempt to explore her emotions more deeply, I encouraged her to depict "her tired" through art. Susan created an image of a woman with yellow swirls emanating from her stomach and extending throughout her body.

I asked her if she had any pain in her stomach and she said no. Despite that, I suggested she consult her primary doctor for a comprehensive check-up to rule out any underlying medical concerns. Several weeks later, Susan returned to our session with tears in her eyes as she revealed her diagnosis of stage one stomach cancer. She explained that the early detection allowed for swift treatment.

Susan's conscious awareness had indicated that something was amiss within her body, but it was only when she delved into her subconscious through art that she could pinpoint the specific nature of her illness. This experience illustrates the profound potential of creative expression in uncovering latent truths about our well-being.

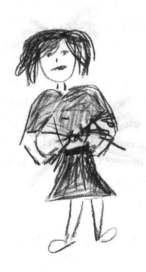

- *Art can provide a means of coping with frustration and disappointment* during the creative process. Life is full of challenges that can lead to negative emotions, but it's important to choose how we respond. Instead of resorting to self-destructive habits like substance abuse, overeating, or withdrawing from others, we can sit with these unpleasant feelings and recognize that they are temporary. Making art offers an opportunity to practice being in a difficult emotional space without serious consequences.

- *Art-making can boost self-esteem and confidence when the final product aligns with, or exceeds, one's initial vision.* The completion of a project, from start to finish, elicits a sense of accomplishment that empowers the individual. This can reduce fears of the unknown and inspire people to tackle new and challenging ventures. The satisfaction derived from creating something that meets one's expectations reinforces a positive self-image and can lead to increased self-assurance.

CCTM combines Art Therapy and Cognitive Behavioral Therapy, two powerful techniques, in a unique way which provides a comprehensive and holistic approach to personal growth and transformation. By integrating the benefits of both CBT and Art Therapy, CCTM offers a transformative process toward healing and self-discovery.

Each session is carefully structured, making this an easy-to-follow format for both therapists and individuals seeking guidance in taking control of their lives. By the end of this introduction, you will have a clear understanding of the unique components that make up each module and how they work together to facilitate personal growth and healing!

NOTES FOR THERAPISTS: USING THIS WORKBOOK TO ENHANCE OR SUPPLEMENT THERAPY

The CCTM is created to be done in 10 sessions. Each Module will correspond to one 50-minute therapy session.

To ensure that your clients get the maximum benefit from this program, I strongly encourage you, yourself, to complete the entire Creative Cognitive Therapy Method. This way, you'll become well-acquainted with all the modules and exercises before introducing them to others. It's possible that this firsthand experience may even lead to improvements in your own well-being throughout the process. Who knows, you might discover some hidden fears that need addressing and you might gain new ways to care for yourself. Being human is hard, and we could all use a little assistance now and then.

When you start using the Creative Cognitive Therapy Method with your clients, it's a good idea to give them a special, blank sketchbook. This way, all their drawings and writings are kept together in one place, making it easier for you both to work with. It's best to use a sketchbook that's about the size of a standard letter paper or even larger. This provides plenty of space for them to draw and express themselves freely. If the sketchbook is too small, it might make them feel cramped, and they might not put as much effort into their drawings. Alternatively, you can also suggest that clients bring their own notebook to the first session if they prefer.

It's a good idea for them to draw directly in the sketch-book. But if you or your client prefer using separate sheets of paper, you can use those clear plastic sleeves that go in a ring binder to keep all the drawings and writings organized.

Foundational information

Before delving into the framework of the Creative Cognitive Therapy Method, let's first explore the fundamental concept of change. The process of personal growth is a journey that many people undertake at some point in their lives. This journey often involves navigating five distinct stages of change. Understanding these stages can be beneficial, as it provides insight into the learning process, and helps to overcome obstacles or setbacks that may arise along the way.

This concept was initially developed by Prochaska and

DiClemente in the late 1970s.[3] I believe it's crucial to grasp why the process of change can often prove to be quite challenging.

Identifying the stages of change
Precontemplation
The first stage of change is the Precontemplation Stage, where we are not yet aware of the need for change. We may be in denial about what the issue is or simply unaware of its existence.

For instance, Madison is in a stressed-out funk—she's experiencing persistent dread and panic attacks. Madison is feeling weighed down by something, but she has not yet taken any steps to uncover what that something is. In fact, at this point she may not even be aware of the impact that her stress is having on her well-being. She has not made a conscious connection between her stress and her health, and therefore she doesn't feel motivated to make any changes in her life. This may also be affecting her relationships.

This first stage is characterized by a lack of awareness or denial that there is even a problem in the first place. This is not yet the point where we seek help or even want change. It can be a difficult stage to confront but accepting that you have been feeling a certain way for a long time is the first step toward a better future. The Precontemplation stage is when we start to acknowledge that something needs to change—that things cannot stay the way they are. When we experience significant distress, whether it's physical or emotional, we are compelled to seek ways to stop that suffering. This is what moves us toward the next stage of change.

Contemplation
The second stage is the Contemplation Stage, a time when we begin to consider change but are not yet fully committed to it. We may be weighing the pros and cons of taking action. Going back to our example of Madison: she now realizes that she needs to reduce her daily stress, because it's making her life unmanageable. But change is scary, and it is hard for Madison to find her

motivation. Madison recognizes that she could probably benefit from a regular exercise routine, but she's having trouble getting started. She keeps making excuses, like not having enough time or money to go to the gym regularly. She may also be considering reaching out for help in the form of therapy, but she's not ready to commit to that quite yet either. Madison is starting to feel frustrated with herself, but she's not given up yet. It's important to note that people may spend a significant amount of time in this stage as they work to overcome their fears and doubts and build their confidence. Anyone can overcome these challenges and move forward toward the next stage of the change journey. In some instances, the path may be smoother with the aid of support and guidance, be it from a compassionate friend, a dedicated therapist, an experienced coach, or even through the utilization of this Creative Cognitive Therapy Method!

Preparation

In the Preparation Stage, we are finally ready to take action toward our desired change. We've weighed the pros and cons and have made a decision to commit to our goals. Going back to Madison: she has now researched the different options available to her and has decided to start a regular exercise routine. She's found a gym that's affordable and conveniently located. She has even purchased some new workout clothes. By taking these small but important steps, Madison is building the momentum and motivation she needs to move forward. It's important to note that this stage may be challenging. We may encounter obstacles and setbacks along the way. But by staying focused on our goals and keeping a positive mindset, we can overcome these challenges and continue to make progress toward the next stage of the change journey.

Action

In the previous stage, Madison decided to reduce stress and is now ready to take action toward her goal. The Action Stage is where we start making tangible changes in our behavior. For Madison, this means she's starting to implement her plan to reduce stress through exercise. She is going to the gym and taking walks regularly and is also incorporating healthy habits into her daily routine. For example, she sets aside a specific time each day for meditation. It's important to maintain focus on the ultimate goal and stay committed to the changes being made during this stage. By consistently making small but meaningful improvements, we can continue to build momentum and achieve our desired outcomes. The Action stage can sometimes bring its own set of challenges and setbacks, but with a willingness to adapt to make necessary adjustments, we can continue moving forward toward lasting change.

Maintenance

The final stage is the Maintenance Stage, where individuals are working to maintain their changes and prevent relapsing back into old behaviors. The journey toward personal growth and development is a continuous process and you may revisit any of these stages multiple times.

Now that exercise is a regular, intentional part of her life, Madison has a deeper sense of self-confidence, self-respect, and capability to handle life's ups and downs. Of course, like anyone else, she may still experience stressors and the blows of life, but she is able to identify them—and control her reactions to them. She is able to use the emotional and physical tools that she sharpened during her journey to sustain inner strength when the inevitable emotional waves of life arise.

What to expect: CCTM module layout

First off, before you embark on your journey with the Creative Cognitive Therapy Method, it's important to gather the materials necessary for a successful experience. I highly recommend investing in a sturdy, hardcover sketchbook, where you can conveniently keep all your drawings and writings together in one place.

Now, here is how the book is set-up (your transformation roadmap):

A relevant quotation

I love a good quotation. Having a quotation at the start of each session sets the tone for a meaningful and impactful conversation. It can also give you a tool to hold onto and be a reminder of your own journey and growth. Quotations often encapsulate powerful concepts related to growth mindset, resilience, gratitude, and self-belief. By regularly exposing ourselves to such quotations, we gradually internalize these empowering beliefs and incorporate them into our mindset. This mindset shift can lead to long-lasting positive changes in our thoughts, behaviors, and overall well-being.

NOTES FOR THERAPISTS

At the beginning of each therapy session, read the quotation to your client and have them write it in their notebook. This makes it easy for your client to look back at the quotation whenever they want. Your clients may also want to write additional comments or thoughts regarding the quotation.

Setting specific goals

To make the most of your mental health journey, it helps to set goals and make an action plan with achievable outcomes that you can realistically implement in your life. With each step you take you will feel a bit more in control of your life, and empowered to keep moving forward by making changes that will help you reach your desired results. It's important to be open and honest with yourself in order to have clarity when working to create your highest self (and life!).

Setting specific goals during each stage of change is a critical step in the personal growth and development process. Therefore, in the next segment, I will be introducing the specific goals that are predetermined for each module. Regularly setting and working toward achievable goals can help increase motivation and a sense of accomplishment, which is beneficial for individuals looking to make positive changes in their lives.

NOTES FOR THERAPISTS

These are the goals for each therapeutic session and how they relate to the stages of change:

Precontemplation Stage goals should help the client:

1. acknowledge a problem that is negatively impacting their life, health, or relationships

2. accept that change is necessary

3. recognize that the current way of doing things is not sustainable in the long run.

Contemplation Stage goals should help the client:

1. access the pros and cons of the current behavior

2. identify potential barriers to change

3. increase self-awareness around the behavior that needs to be changed

4. consider the impact of the behavior or situation on one's self and others around them.

Preparation Stage goals should help the client:

1. be able to research and gather information about different options available for achieving change

2. seek out support and guidance from others who have successfully achieved a similar change

3. make necessary preparations to remove potential barriers to successful change.

Action Stage goals should help the client:

1. consistently engage in new behavior

2. monitor progress and make adjustments as needed

3. create a support system to help stay motivated and accountable

4. build confidence and self-efficiency by recognizing progress and accomplishments.

Maintenance Stage goals should help the client:

1. continue to practice new habits and behaviors consistently

2. practice self-reflection to monitor progress and build self-awareness

3. celebrate achievements along the way

4. plan and have strategies in place for potential obstacles.

Cognitive Behavioral Therapy (CBT)

The CBT intervention is an important part of the session as it aims to challenge and change negative or irrational thought patterns that may be contributing to the individual's problem. By identifying and challenging cognitive distortions, individuals can gain a more accurate and positive perspective on themselves and their experiences. This can lead to reduced feelings of anxiety, depression, and other negative emotions, and can improve overall mental health and well-being. This process helps to solidify the insights gained during the session and encourages the individual to continue making progress toward their goals.

> ## NOTES FOR THERAPISTS
> Guide your clients to record the CBT exercise responses in their sketchbook. Following this, they can either read aloud what they've written to you, or if they prefer, initiate a discussion about their answers. If a conversation precedes the written summary, they can jot down a brief recap of the CBT exercise in their sketchbook afterward. In either approach, keeping the CBT exercises in their notebook enhances the overall program's continuity and equips them with the capability to revisit completed exercises as needed.

Art Therapy

The use of Art Therapy tools follows Cognitive Behavioral Therapy (CBT) exercises, providing a complementary and alternative form of expression. You'll require a variety of drawing materials in multiple colors. This can include crayons, colored pens, colored pencils, and markers, among others. Additionally, you'll need other art supplies like watercolor paints, a paintbrush, colored paper, scissors, tape, and glue. These materials don't have to be expensive or top-of-the-line; whatever you have available will suffice.

Some exercises use material that can be downloaded for your own use at www.jkp.com/catalogue/book/9781805011590, as indicated by a ✪ symbol.

> ## NOTES FOR THERAPISTS
> No matter whether the client is drawing directly in the sketchbook or on loose paper kept in a binder, make sure there is one consistent place to keep all the drawings. This

provides a safe place for their artwork. In addition, it gives a sense that the art and the writing that they are doing have a chronological process. It shows respect for all the work your clients are doing throughout the entire program.

While the client is creating art, it's common for therapists to feel as though they might be making their clients uncomfortable by simply observing them draw or paint. But often clients become deeply engrossed in the artistic process and may not pay attention to your presence. I encourage you to embrace the silence, allowing your clients to concentrate. Pay attention to how your client interacts with the art materials. Are they eager to start, or do they approach it hesitantly? What colors do they choose? Do they invest significant time erasing and starting over, or can they accept mistakes? These observations offer valuable insights into your client's personality and how they engage with their world.

Explanation and discussion prompts

Many individuals hold limiting beliefs about their own creativity and artistic abilities, often due to negative experiences in school or early childhood. The labeling of art as an elective, and lack of exposure to the essential skills required for creating successful artwork, can cause individuals to abandon art-making at a young age. I encourage anyone who feels that they are "not good at art" to participate in Art Therapy. This is because, for those who don't consider themselves artists, becoming familiar with lines, shapes, and colors as a "language" can lead to a more uninhibited self-expression, enabling deeper exploration of their subconscious. After the Art Therapy exercise, a reflective discussion takes place. The use of thought-provoking questions and prompts helps to delve deeper into the symbolism and emotions embodied in the artwork. Individuals can choose to document their insights through writing, journaling, or by discussing them with a trusted friend, mentor, or therapist. This step further enhances the therapeutic benefits of the Art Therapy process by promoting self-reflection and promoting deeper understanding.

NOTES FOR THERAPISTS

Take the time to talk with your clients about the purpose of doing the specific exercise and how it will benefit them.

Your clients don't need to write down their answers to the discussion prompts. These prompts are more of a general guide to help you have a chat about the Art Therapy exercises after they've completed them.

Additional exercises, follow up, and next steps
Finally, the last section includes additional assignments to build upon the insights gained and prepare for the next session.

NOTES FOR THERAPISTS

Use these additional exercises as homework so they can keep working on the CCTM progress between therapy sessions. Encourage them to keep these assignments in the same sketchbook or folder where they are keeping their other work. This way, everything, including the homework, works together to help your clients make progress in their personal growth.

When they come back for the next therapy session, set aside a little time to review the homework and discuss anything new that's popped up since your last meeting.

In this book, the names and identifying details of individuals have been altered to protect their privacy. Each story you will encounter is rooted in real experiences, but I have taken care to change specific information to ensure the anonymity of my clients. This approach allows me to share the valuable lessons and insights gleaned from their journeys while respecting their confidentiality. Rest assured, the essence of their stories remains intact, providing authentic and meaningful narratives that reflect the true spirit of their experiences.

This program is structured into 10 modules, each building on the knowledge and skills gained in the previous one, to guide you through a comprehensive journey of self-improvement. Each chapter corresponds to an entire module, and each module consistently adheres to the comprehensive five-part format explained earlier.

The whole program is designed to tackle deep-seated issues and equip you with effective coping mechanisms. You will gain a deeper understanding of your thoughts, beliefs, and behaviors, and learn to adopt healthier responses to life's challenges, such as anxiety, irritability, depression, or anger. Are you ready to embark on a transformative journey that will help you see yourself in a new light? Let's go!

First Module:
Beginning Your Journey —Where Are You?

The world outside is teeming with factors beyond our control. However, when we purposefully dedicate ourselves to fostering positive changes within, we enhance our capacity to react with resilience and inner tranquility to the people and circumstances we can neither change nor control. As the poet Rumi succinctly expressed, *"Yesterday, I was clever, so I wanted to change the world. Today, I am wise, so I am changing myself."*[4] This quotation serves as a compelling reminder that personal growth and development is really the only control we have.

Goal: What do you want to change?

This section is about asking yourself who you are, where you are, and identifying what you want to change.

You might find it helpful to write out your responses in your journal to the following questions for future reference.

1. Who are you? Not just your job but also your passions, your dreams, your relationships, and your fears.

2. How has your own culture influenced you, your choices, and your lifestyle (in positive and negative ways)?

3. What do you want to change in your life?

4. What are you willing to do differently?

5. What are you willing to give up?

CBT intervention: Baby Steps

If you believe that small steps are insignificant, then you will never take any steps toward growth. But if you believe that every step counts, and you take one small step every day for a year, then you will have taken 365 steps. A year from now you will be in a whole different place. The Baby Steps concept is based on the idea that when attempting any challenging task, it is beneficial to break it down into manageable pieces. The concept encourages us to focus on taking small, gradual steps toward our goals. This approach allows us to easily conquer any challenge by focusing on just one step at a time, instead of feeling overwhelmed by an entire task or project.

My client Joshua wanted to improve his financial state.

I asked him: "What is one small step you will take today to be in a better place a year from now?"

He said: "I will start to track my spending and create a realistic budget."

He decided to set aside $10 per week to put into savings. After a few months he was able to increase that $10 to $25. Additionally, he began to research investments, such as stocks and mutual funds, to learn more about other ways to increase his wealth.

Question: What is one small step *you* will take today to be in a better place a year from now? Spend some time thinking about this and write out your answer.

Art Therapy exercise: Draw a bridge

For this Art Therapy exercise, I am going to ask you to draw a bridge. It can be a real or made-up bridge. It can be something that you have seen in real life or in a photo or a movie. Or something that totally comes from your own imagination. Your bridge can be made from traditional bridge materials, for example, wood, stone, or metal. Or your bridge can be made from fantasy materials such as balloons, clouds, or anything else you are inspired to draw. It can be going from any one place to any other place. Lastly, use whatever colors you want and add any additional elements to make your bridge look as creative as you would like. Upon completing the bridge drawing, position yourself within the scene. You have the creative freedom to draw a person or simply mark your location with a dot or an X. Take a moment to reflect and make a conscious choice: Will you place yourself on the bridge, beside it, or underneath it? Consider whether you are in motion or at a standstill. If you're in motion, you can enhance your depiction with a small arrow to signify the direction of your movement. This exercise invites you to engage your imagination and explore your emotions through your artistic choices.

Explanation and discussion prompts

The Art Therapy exercise "Draw a bridge" holds within it a rich tapestry of metaphors that can deeply resonate with individuals undergoing various life challenges. The most obvious metaphor here is "transition." Picture a bridge, and you'll see why. Bridges are all about moving from one place to another. You start in one place and journey to another. Is the person who begins on one side of the bridge the same as the person who arrives on the other side?

Drawing a bridge isn't just about sketching; it's a way to express your emotions tied to these transitions. Bridges are constructed to provide stability and assurance as we traverse unfamiliar terrain. The bridge drawings often reveal how safe or unsafe one feels in the world. Through this exercise, you can reflect on how it feels to be on a bridge and what would make you feel more secure. The idea of a bridge extends to that of a "support system." Just as a bridge relies on its pillars and structure for strength, we can use this exercise to explore our own support networks. It's not uncommon for individuals I work with to craft bridges that appear to hover in mid-air, seemingly unsupported. When this observation arises, it frequently prompts them to open up about their feelings of inadequacy or a perceived absence of support in their lives. Consider what is supporting the bridge. How could the bridge represent your support system?

Another metaphor to consider is related to movement within your drawing. Ask yourself if you appear stationary or in motion. Does it reflect how you feel in your life—as if you're stuck or making progress? If you're in the midst of a transition, consider whether you're at the beginning, middle, or end of it. Alternatively, perhaps you're moving backward, retracing your steps toward something from your past.

Spend some time with the following questions. These can serve as valuable prompts for engaging in reflective journal writing, enabling you to delve even deeper into the exercises. If you are collaborating with a therapist or coach, these questions can form a basis for insightful discussions. Feel free to explore the questions in any order that resonate with you. There's no obligation to respond to all of them. Their purpose is to spark meaningful conversations and encourage introspection.

- What feelings or thoughts did you experience while drawing the bridge?

- What memories does this bridge bring up for you?

- What do you think bridges symbolize for you?

- What is holding your bridge up? And how does that relate or represent your personal social support system?

- Are you moving or standing still?

- – If you are moving, what direction are you moving in? Left to right? Right to left? Diagonally? Bottom to top? Top to bottom?

- – If you are standing still, what would make you/force you to move?

- How would it feel to cross this bridge?

  - – Would it feel safe or unsafe?

  - – What would make you feel safer?

- What do you think the bridge represents in your life?

- What is on either side of the bridge?

  - – How are those sides different or the same?

- What are you going toward/coming from?

- What transition in your life does this bridge represent?

To provide a more engaging and immersive learning experience with the Creative Cognitive Therapy Method, I want to share a real-life case study with you. So, let's dive right in and see what it's like for both Erin and me to embark on this transformative journey together.

ERIN'S STORY

The young woman was obviously anxious, but she possessed an air of self-confidence as she walked into the room. She presented as a healthy woman, dressed in expensive-looking yoga clothes. She mentioned that her first language was Spanish, which told me that her cultural background was important to her and she wanted me to know that it was part of her whole self.

"My name is Erin. I'm 24 years old and I'm a personal trainer. I'm here because I have anxiety issues that I'm hoping to address through this program." I could tell she was ready to take the first step toward healing. "I'm so glad you're here. I understand how difficult this can be," I said, creating a safe and accepting environment. "I'm here to help you. I have extensive experience with CBT and Art Therapy, and I'm confident that with the Creative Cognitive Therapy Method you'll be able to make significant progress in the next 10 weeks. I'm here to provide the guidance, support, and direction you need, and I'll do my best to make sure your journey is positive, enjoyable, and productive. I ask you to show up consistently, be open-minded about doing things outside your comfort zone, and between our sessions, complete the homework assignments and practice the tools that you learn."

She settled back further into the chair and shared that she was really excited about this because she had never done Art Therapy before. In fact, she never even knew that Art Therapy existed until she spoke to me. I was excited for her. She began to relax even more and told me that, despite the fact that her job was teaching others the importance of healthy living, she often neglected this for herself. She was regularly not getting enough rest and not eating healthy food, and she felt guilty about it. I noticed Erin started to use the pronoun "you" when she was actually referring to her own behaviors. For instance, she said, "Maybe you didn't eat right that day, or maybe you stayed up too late the night before." Feelings of guilt and shame are frequently linked to disordered eating behaviors, suggesting a possible emotional struggle regarding their relationship with food. I decided to keep that in mind and see if it would come up again in other contexts.

In my experience, when someone says "you" when referring to their own behaviors, they are not taking responsibility or ownership of their actions. Instead of saying "I," they are using the third-person point of view to distance themselves from the situation. This can be seen as a form of avoidance or deflection and can signal evasion of accountability.

Erin expressed that as a personal trainer, she put a lot of pressure on herself to be perfect. I could totally relate, and I disclosed that being a therapist can have a lot of pressure to be perfect also. By revealing my own insecurities, I was building trust.

Then I asked Erin to talk about her anxiety, and she said, "I was doing okay, but in the last few weeks it feels like I have fallen into a deep hole. I've been motivating everyone around me except myself." Erin explained that she had a bachelor's degree in health and fitness, but she felt quite anxious about what her future should look like.

We discussed the different goals Erin wanted to accomplish in therapy, which included creating healthier sleep and eating routines, reducing anxiety, and gaining clarity about what she wanted for her future such as graduate school, work, and/or a potential move.

I asked Erin if she was ready to make some art, and she expressed insecurity about her artistic abilities. I explained that we all have an inner critical voice; I actually refer to mine as "my opponent." I encouraged her to acknowledge that inner critic, but not to let it get in the way of making art. This emphasized the importance of allowing herself to explore her creativity, despite any doubts or preconceived ideas that might be present.

I instructed Erin to draw a bridge.

Erin hesitated but slowly picked up a dark blue marker and started to draw. At first, she found it hard to focus, but after a few times she became more confident and willing to take on the challenge. When she was nearing the end of her drawing, I directed Erin to place herself somewhere in the drawing.

Even though she had asked if she could use any color, her bridge was monochromatic, all drawn in dark blue. It seemed that she did not want to spend too much time drawing. Maybe she felt uncomfortable or maybe she was concerned that I would be bored by waiting for her to finish. I asked Erin if she would like to add any other colors, and she said, "I will add some more colors and make it prettier." She drew for several more minutes, adding colors and chatting openly with me about her life and her work.

Her bridge was floating in space, and made up of many tiny, little squares, which she described as bricks. A tree was perched on either side of the bridge. Above the bridge were three upside-down V's, which Erin said represented birds. Below the bridge were nine similar upside-down V's, that she described as a body of water. She said that she was trying to create a tranquil and meditative environment.

Erin drew herself on the far-right side of the bridge, and when I asked her if she was moving or standing still in this drawing, she described herself as standing still, but if she were to eventually move, it would be to the left.

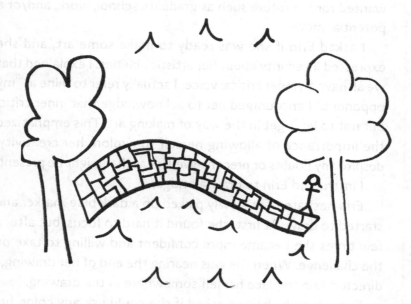

We then had an open dialogue, led by the discussion prompts. Erin had drawn a bridge that was floating, not grounded or supported. Erin's metaphor of this bridge was that everything was up in the air, and she felt as though she did not have much support. I pointed out, and Erin agreed, that the birds in the sky probably symbolized the most prominent people in her family: her mother, her father, her brother, and herself. As we were talking, she decided to add color and more birds to the sky. Erin acknowledged that she was open to the possibility of more people coming into her life.

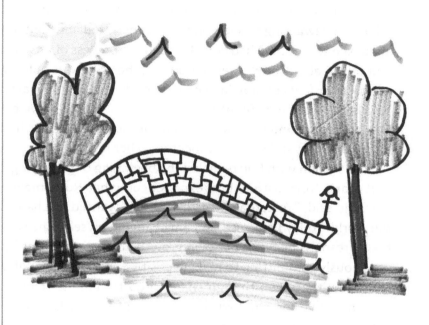

Erin described the figure as moving from right to left. I asked Erin if it felt like the figure in the drawing was moving forward or backward, and she quickly responded that it definitely felt like she was moving backward. I agreed with her and explained that because in our society we read from left to right, our brains are programmed to recognize this direction as a forward movement, and hence moving from right to left feels like a backwards movement. We talked about her having just crossed over the bridge and maybe turning around and going back toward the other side from where she just came.

I asked her, "Is there anything in your life that you have just completed, and you are about to go back to?" She laughed and said, "I have been thinking about going back to school to get my graduate degree."

As we wrapped up the first session, Erin remarked, "That was fun and calming. I loved it!" She was amazed at how a simple drawing could reveal so much. As she left my office, I felt confident that our next session would be even more successful. It was rewarding to see Erin feeling energized and content about the session. We had gone through the process of artwork and talked about how it resonated with her. She was able to get past her fears of drawing and create a bridge that revealed parallels to her own life. At the end of the session, I provided Erin with the homework assignment of journaling about her bridge drawing and how it connected to her life.

The session with Erin revealed the beginning of real change that starts from within. Erin experienced what Rumi meant when he said, "Yesterday I was clever, so I wanted to change the world. Today I am wise, so I am changing myself." She was taking responsibility for her own growth and development by consciously committing to making positive changes in her life. She knew that even though she desired to help her clients become healthier, she had to help herself first. It felt like a successful accomplishment.

NOTES FOR THERAPISTS

The aim of this first therapy session is to establish a strong foundation by getting to know your new client and understanding their true challenges. On the other hand, if you've been working with this client for some time, your objective shifts to assisting them in identifying and concentrating on the specific areas in their life that they wish to enhance and change.

In this first session, lead your client through the CBT exercise, "Baby Steps." Use the discussion prompts to open up a dialogue about change. Encourage your client to jot down a few notes to reference back to later. Alternatively, they can write it all out in their journal, but be aware that will take up more of your session time.

Then move directly into the Art Therapy exercise. When a new client first sees the art supplies, I like to give them options. For example, I might ask, "Do you want to use crayons, colored pencils, or markers?"

I also let the client decide how they want to position the paper, whether horizontally or vertically. I'll mention that they can turn the paper any way they like for their drawing. Sometimes, clients who are not used to making art might not even realize they have these choices, so it's good to point them out. It helps them feel more comfortable and in control of the process.

As your client draws, pay attention to how they do it without interrupting. It can actually tell you a lot about how they handle things in their everyday life. The way they make art often reflects how they approach many other situations. Keep an eye out for whether they dive into drawing with excitement, or if they seem hesitant or get easily frustrated. Later, you can mention these observations and ask if they've faced similar situations lately where they've reacted in a similar way. It's a way to understand them better

Sometimes, you might feel like you need to talk or ask questions to fill the silence, but you don't have to. Let them be in the moment of drawing. However, if they start talking while they're drawing, of course, you can respond and have a regular conversation.

At the end of the first session, ask them to journal about their bridge as a homework assignment. Below are the prompts you can suggest they explore.

• Describe the colors, shapes and images.

- Ask the bridge where it is taking you.

- Ask yourself: where do you want to go?

- Who or what would make you move?

- What are you leaving and what are you going toward?

- How are the two sides of the bridge different/same?

Remind your client to do their journaling in the same sketchbook or folder, so everything stays in one place. Encourage them to bring this sketchbook or folder with them to the next therapy session. Lastly, tell your client that you are proud of them for showing up today and having the courage to be willing to dig deep and make changes to improve their mental well-being.

CHAPTER TWO

Second Module:
What is Holding You Back?

Once you have identified a particular issue or problem in your life, you have the responsibility to either accept it as it is or take real steps toward changing it. By taking ownership of a challenge in your life, you are actively working to address it. The quotation below emphasizes the importance of self-awareness and accountability. You are now ready to stake a claim to your own issues or problems. Although I have no idea who originally said it, this statement rings true to me: *"Once you name it, you must claim it."*

Goals: What do you want to work on?

The goals for Module Two are to identify your primary challenge, whether it's fear, anxiety, anger, self-esteem, or another issue, and to prepare yourself for the process of making meaningful change. These goals are about really getting to the core of what brought you here today. Understanding the core issue provides you with clarity and a deeper understanding of what truly troubles you beyond surface-level symptoms. This understanding allows you to implement targeted solutions that address the root cause, leading to lasting transformation.

Let's take a look at the case of my client, Luisa, who had been in a relationship with Patrick for four-and-a-half years. Their arguments had become frequent and intense. She'd started to feel disconnected from him and harbored a growing resentment.

If Luisa solely focused on the specific arguments, she only found temporary solutions to alleviate the conflicts, which ended up being superficial and short-lived. She was frustrated that therapy was not working.

Once Luisa dove into her core issues, which were centered around the struggle she had with her own self-esteem and poor boundaries, she gradually experienced a positive shift in her relationship with Patrick. By prioritizing her own well-being, she became more assertive in expressing her needs and concerns, leading to improved communication and a greater sense of connection. The changes she made were not merely surface level, but transformative and sustainable. This shift had a positive effect not only on her relationship with Patrick, but on all her personal and professional interactions.

So, how do you identify your core issue? You need to take a moment and ask yourself:

1. What is causing stress in your life?

2. What is interfering with your work/career?

    - Is there anything deeper or underlying that might be contributing?

3. What is damaging your relationships?

    - Is there anything deeper or underlying that might be contributing?

4. What is affecting your health and well-being?

    - Is there anything deeper or underlying that might be contributing?

5. What do you need to change?

CBT intervention: Tune in

It is a common belief that our thoughts have control over us. While this may be true for many individuals, it doesn't have to be the case for everyone. We all experience automatic negative thoughts (ANTs) that infest our minds and attempt to influence our perception of reality. But here's the empowering truth: You have the ability to decide which thoughts you want to embrace and which ones are nothing but, well, total nonsense.

By actively listening to your thoughts and becoming aware of their presence, you can gain a sense of control over them. Rather than automatically assuming that every thought crossing your mind is true, you have the power to question the validity of each one and assess how it affects your well-being. This process of careful consideration empowers you to distinguish between reality and imagination, enabling you to consciously select which thoughts you want to welcome into your mind.

I will give you a very personal example: I've often struggled with imposter syndrome as a Jewish bisexual woman. Although I try to be engaged in both the Jewish and LGBTQ+ communities, I frequently feel like I am not enough of either identity and I don't truly belong, which has left me feeling disconnected.

My negative thoughts sound like "I don't speak Hebrew, and I've never been to Israel, so I can't be a 'real' Jew" or "I am married to a man so I can pass as heterosexual and I'm not queer enough." These thoughts have deepened my feelings of not fitting in, and for many years I pulled away from both communities, believing that I didn't meet the criteria to be considered a true member.

To combat these feelings of inadequacy, I've started to challenge my negative thoughts. Instead of fixating on what I lack, I try to embrace my unique journey as a Jewish bisexual woman. I've come to understand that there's no one-size-fits-all way to be Jewish or queer. I've realized that my experiences, perspectives, and identity are valid and crucial, no matter how they may differ from others in my communities.

By changing my thoughts to celebrate my individuality, I've

started to feel more connected and confident. I've consciously shifted my focus to thoughts that remind me that I don't just belong here, I also enrich and diversify both communities.

As you take this approach, you transform from a passive recipient of your thoughts into an active participant in your mental landscape. You become a mindful observer, realizing that your thoughts aren't unalterable truths; instead, they are shaped by your beliefs, past experiences, and conditioning. By understanding this, you can intentionally choose thoughts that are supportive, empowering, and aligned with your goals and values.

My client, Andrea, grappled with profound feelings of insecurity and struggles with low self-esteem. She worried about failing at adulthood and not living up to the life she'd expected. Andrea wrestled with the belief that people didn't like her. There was rarely a time when she didn't feel like an imposter at work and in social situations. In our third session together, I asked her to write out a list of her automatic negative thoughts.

Below is a list of her ANTs:

- I am needy.
- I can't speak my mind.
- I will never change.
- I've messed up again.
- I am failing at being an adult.
- I don't have the life I expected.
- People don't like me.

Art Therapy exercise: What you are carrying/holding

This Art Therapy exercise is designed to help you explore and visually represent the burdens, stressors, and emotions that you carry in your life. Envision yourself carrying many objects—these symbolize your automatic negative thoughts (ANTs). Picture yourself grappling with the weight of these burdens. When you've documented five ANTs, visualize yourself supporting each object. Next, choose an image that either contains or symbolizes these burdensome objects. It could be boxes or circles or flowers— something that is easy for you to draw. Now, get your markers, crayons, or paints ready!

1. Begin by drawing a person to represent yourself. This can be as simple as a stick person or more detailed. You can choose any pose or position that feels authentic to you, and not too complicated to draw.

2. Next, imagine yourself holding or carrying many objects. If you chose boxes to represent your ANTs, and wrote five ANTs, you will be holding five boxes.

3. Decide where you want to place the objects in your self-portrait. You could be carrying a tower of ANTs in your hands, on your head, on your back, on your shoulders, or even with your feet.

Back to Andrea. She drew herself as a stick person. She represented her ANTs as a collection of boxes. She chose to depict herself holding three boxes in one hand and two in the other hand. The boxes were unsteady, tipping and teetering, as if about to fall. This may have symbolized the weight and difficulty of carrying these ANTs, suggesting that they were challenging to manage.

Additionally, Andrea drew one box resting precariously on top of her head. The presence of the box on her head represented how her negative thoughts could consume her mind and create an added sense of pressure. Andrea also drew one box that had fallen on her foot. The impact of her ANTs may have been causing her actual physical discomfort and pain.

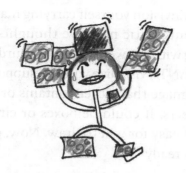

The overall composition of the drawing conveys Andrea's struggle with her ANTs. The falling and unsteady boxes highlighted the difficulties she faced in managing and finding balance amidst these burdens.

Keep in mind that every drawing will be unique, and Andrea's example demonstrates how the chosen object, in this case, boxes, can be incorporated into the self-portrait to represent the ANTs and evoke feelings of instability, burden, and struggle.

Explanation and discussion prompts

After going through the Art Therapy exercises, you may find that you are now able to express your emotions and thoughts in a way you couldn't before. That is why it's really powerful to have a discussion, or journal, immediately following the exercise. These questions are designed to spark meaningful conversations and encourage exploration of different aspects of your drawing and what it represents.

These questions provide an opportunity to express your thoughts, feelings, and experiences when before you may not have words for them. Examine different aspects of your drawing and your inner world. It may enhance self-awareness, metaphors, and deeper insight. Get out your journal and explore the following questions:

1. What are you holding?

2. How does it feel to hold all those things at once?

3. Is the load heavy or awkward?

4. What are you not able to do because you are holding so many things?

5. What could you do if your hands weren't full?

6. Would you be willing to let go of any?

7. Which ones seem heavier/lighter than others?

8. How does your drawing reflect your current experiences or challenges in life?

ERIN'S STORY

Erin depicted herself as a stick figure precariously leaning to the left, suggesting instability and a sense of almost falling. The figure appears to be floating, disconnected from the ground, emphasizing a lack of grounding. The expression on her face is flat and emotionless, and the entire drawing is monochromatic. These elements poignantly reflect her current state, all of which will evolve and transform as Erin progresses through this program. Erin made the creative choice to represent each of her ANTs as a different symbol. Instead of holding onto all of them, they were all floating around her. When I asked Erin about this, she said "I guess everything is just up in the air right now." Erin had identified her ANTs as:

- I don't know who I am.

- I don't know what my future holds.

- Time is running out.

- I need to get a master's degree.

- I stay up too late.

- Sometimes I over-exercise.

- Should I move?

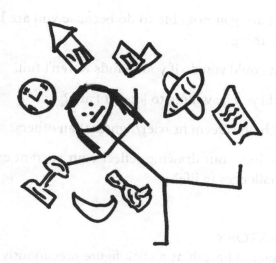

Additional exercises, follow up, and next steps: Get those ANTs out of your PANTs

At the beginning of our session, you wrote a list of ANTs (Automatic Negative Thoughts). Remember that old saying "You've got ants in your pants?" It meant that you were restless and couldn't sit still. Personally, the association between ants and pants remains etched in my mind. Therefore, I've created the acronym PANTs, signifying Present Affirming Nurturing Thoughts. This encapsulates the notion of steering thoughts toward a positive and nurturing self. Because most of our ANTs tend to focus on catastrophizing the future or regretting the past, it is vital to keep your PANTs in the now. Unlike movie *The Sisterhood of the Traveling Pants*, make sure your PANTs stick to the now and resist the urge to wander off into the past or future! (If you're not familiar with the reference, I recommend the book or the movie!) For example, if the ANT is "I can't accomplish my goals," the corresponding PANT would be "I am achieving my goals."

It's important to understand that you do not have to believe your PANTs. The key is just recognizing that there's an alternative perspective. We can never fully rid ourselves of the ANTs, but we can, and must, learn to balance all those self-deprecating internal statements with positive affirmations. Remember, you do not have to believe the statement. Just write it down, despite the fact that it sounds like a lie. These new PANTs feel uncomfortable and don't fit right because we have spent considerable time reinforcing the negative self-talk, thereby ingraining those pessimistic thoughts into automatic responses. Similar to how repeated exposure to advertising can influence our beliefs, the constant infestation of ANTs has reinforced their hold on us. We can challenge and replace these negative beliefs, by putting on your big-person PANTs!

Therefore, throughout the week, listen for any new ANTs, and add them to your list. But for each ANT you write, you must also write a PANT. This will be a statement that is the exact opposite.

One more thing, and this is important, you must find a time of the day when you can say the PANTs to yourself. It will only take you about 60 seconds, but it makes a world of difference. Make this a routine, which will eventually turn into a habit. Remember all PANTs must be both positive and in the present tense.

Returning to the example of Andrea, here is her list of ANTs and PANTs. Notice how she keeps the PANTs simple and in the present tense.

ANTs	PANTs
I am needy.	I rely on others for support.
I can't speak my mind.	I do speak my mind.
I will never change.	I am constantly changing.
I've messed up again.	I am successful.
I am failing at being an adult.	I am an adult.

I don't have the life I expected.	I am living my life.
People don't like me.	People like me.

The fascinating aspect is that both the ANTs (Automatic Negative Thought) and the PANTs (Present Affirming New Thoughts) can coexist at the same time. They are both valid perspectives and neither is truer than the other.

For instance, Andrea does display signs of neediness in specific situations or with certain individuals, yet she also exhibits independence in various aspects of her life. While it may be true that some people don't like Andrea, it is equally true that many people genuinely like and even love her. This exercise doesn't involve feigning an overly positive or idealistic outlook, but rather recognizing that any thought can have two sides to it.

By actively challenging and replacing negative thoughts with positive and present-focused alternatives, you take an empowered stance in reshaping your mindset. Through self-awareness and a commitment to personal growth, you pave the way for greater resilience, improved self-perception, and a more fulfilling life. Remember, the journey to adopting PANTs is a transformative process that unfolds over time, and each step forward brings us closer to a more positive and empowering mindset.

Creating a dedicated time each day to practice saying the PANTs to yourself can be incredibly beneficial. I suggest incorporating this practice into your morning routine, maybe while brushing your teeth. By doing so, you will establish a consistent habit and set a positive tone for the day ahead. Consistency is crucial, as it helps reinforce the new thought patterns you are cultivating. As you repeatedly affirm these positive thoughts, you will begin to internalize them, gradually replacing the negative narratives you have carried for so long.

Over the upcoming week, make a conscious effort to remain vigilant for any additional ANTs that might be running through your mind. Whenever you identify these negative thoughts, promptly add them to your list and work on substituting them with PANTs. Integrate the new PANTs into your daily morning routine. Maintain this practice consistently for several consecutive days. After about a week, take a moment to reflect by asking yourself the following questions:

1. Were there any challenges to creating the PANTs?

2. Did you actually make time every day to say your PANTs? Why or why not?

3. If you did:

   a. How did that feel?

   b. Did your belief of those statements shift at all?

   c. Did it become easier or harder each day?

   d. Did you notice that it changed your mood, your choices, or your interactions with others?

4. If you did not:

   a. How did that feel?

   b. What stopped you or got in your way?

   c. What were the new ANTs that arose as obstacles to the activity? (E.g., "I don't have time," "It won't make a difference," "This is stupid"...)

   d. Write new PANTs for those.

The journey from thoughts to actions to habits to character is profound. Thoughts, when nurtured and focused upon, manifest into actions—both positive and negative. With repetition and consistency, these actions solidify into habits, becoming ingrained patterns of behavior that shape our daily lives. Our character emerges as the sum total of our thoughts and actions, affects how we perceive the world, how we interact with others, and ultimately, how we navigate life. Therefore, it is crucial to cultivate a conscious awareness of our thoughts, for they possess the power to shape not only our actions but also the very essence of who we are.

Sit with the questions "Who do I want to be?" and "What character traits do I want people to use when describing me?"

When Maggie first came into therapy she was depressed, isolated, and feeling stuck.

Maggie's ANTs included: "I am lazy," "I am fat," and "I don't deserve to be loved."

Maggie's PANTs included: "I am energetic," "I am healthy," and "I am loved."

If she chose to nourish her ANTs, the repercussions would continue to reverberate throughout her daily routine. The belief of being lazy would take hold, causing her to repeatedly hit the snooze button and oversleep. This might lead to rushed mornings, grabbing a donut as a substitute for breakfast, then spiraling into self-loathing and feeling fat again. This would further undermine her confidence, leading to the perception of being unworthy of love. Convinced that no one could ever find her attractive, she would delete her dating apps and stop dating all together. This would perpetuate the narrative that she was unlovable.

However, an alternative path was before Maggie, one that required embracing the PANTs. And that is what she did! In the beginning it felt silly and disingenuous, but through repetition, she courageously accepted the statements such as "I am energetic," "I am healthy," and "I am loved." She gradually opened herself up to the transformative power of those beliefs.

Through consistent repetition of positive self-talk, Maggie discovered the stark contrast between fleeting, short-term gratification—like hitting the snooze button—and profound, lasting fulfillment that comes from taking care of yourself, fueling your body, and actively participating in life.

This newfound time and energy allowed her to prioritize

exercise and prepare a nutritious breakfast, setting a positive tone for the day ahead. The shift in Maggie's inner narrative created a ripple effect, influencing her choices, actions, and interactions with others. With a renewed sense of self-worth, she eagerly embraced the prospect of meeting people and possibly embarking on new romantic endeavors. By fostering self-love and remaining open to the love of others, Maggie underwent a profound transformation, gradually becoming receptive to joy.

The notion of "Once you name it, you must claim it" underscores the idea that simply identifying negative thoughts is not enough. To effect real change in your life, you must take ownership of them. Having successfully identified detrimental self-talk patterns, it's now imperative to embrace them. These thoughts belong to you, and it's within your power to transform them. This means accepting that these thoughts are a part of your consciousness and it's your responsibility to address them.

NOTES FOR THERAPISTS

After introducing the quotation and objectives for the second therapy session, take a moment to revisit the previously assigned homework, which involved journaling about the bridge drawing. Inquire if your client has any thoughts or insights to share regarding their journaling experience, or if they have made any newfound realizations in their drawing since your initial session together. Dedicate a few minutes to exploring these if necessary.

Use the "Explanation and discussion prompts" to start a conversation after your client has completed their CBT exercise of writing their ANTs (automatic negative thoughts) in the notebook. It is powerful to see all those horrific statements that we say to ourselves. Encourage them to leave a few blank pages between their ANTs and the Art Therapy drawing. That way your client will have space to add any new ANTs that arise between sessions. It also gives them space to write the PANTs (Present Affirming Nurturing Thoughts) as part of their homework.

Also, for homework, encourage your client to invest some time in generating alternative thoughts that can challenge the negative self-talk. Emphasize the importance of keeping these thoughts in the present tense. Additionally, remind your clients that they don't need to fully believe these new thoughts just yet; the exercise is about opening the door to more positive thinking.

Instruct your client to choose a time every day when they will take a few minutes to say these PANTs as affirmations to themselves. Ensure that your clients grasp the importance of incorporating the new PANTs into their daily routine until your next meeting. This allows them to practice and internalize these positive thoughts.

Let your client know that identifying Present Affirming Nurturing Thoughts (PANTs) to replace Automatic Negative Thoughts (ANTs) can sometimes be challenging. Assure them that if they encounter any difficulties, you are there to assist and guide them during your next session.

CHAPTER THREE

Third Module:
Externalize and Face Fears

Art Therapy is highly effective because it encourages us to visualize and express our unconscious thoughts and emotions. Just like turning on a flashlight in a dark room, when we bring these concealed feelings into the light of conscious awareness, they often appear less daunting and lose their grip on us. As I like to say, *"When you can make the unconscious* conscious, *that can dissipate the emotional charge."* In other words, once we confront our hidden emotions, they become less overwhelming, less emotionally charged. I firmly believe that by bringing the unconscious into conscious awareness, whether through verbal expression or artistic representation on paper, one can dissipate the emotional charge these feelings hold over us.

Goals: Get it out

The goals of Module Three are to externalize and confront your fears, followed by the critical step of challenging these fears. This module is designed to empower you to tackle and overcome the obstacles that might be holding you back.

Starting now, I will use the term "your fear" to specifically address the fundamental issue that led you to explore the Creative Cognitive Therapy Method. Everyone has a different struggle and I recognize that you might be grappling with grief while someone else may be primarily dealing with anger. With that said, you might wonder why I choose to use the term "fear" to describe a wide range of issues. It's essential to recognize that the underlying factor driving individuals to seek therapy often traces back to fear.

Let me say that again. Most of what causes us emotional discomfort can be traced back to fear. Take, for instance, my client Rajesh, who sought therapy due to his intense jealousy and overprotectiveness within his marriage. It became evident after just one session that beneath his jealousy, a profound fear lurked: The fear that his wife might find someone more suitable and abandon their relationship. Digging even deeper, we uncovered another layer of fear—the fear of not being deserving of her love.

Another client, Sean, sought therapy to address chronic social anxiety. As we dove into his anxiety, it became evident that his core fear extended beyond public situations. Sean's underlying fear centered on the persistent belief that people would perceive him as unintelligent. This foundational fear was deeply rooted in his self-perception, where he struggled with the notion that he was inherently stupid.

The deep-seated fear for Marissa, who grappled with the trauma of early childhood abuse, was that the world was inherently unsafe, and that she could never trust or feel secure with another person.

This is why this module focuses on identifying and addressing deep-rooted fears. When you can bring these fears to your conscious awareness, either by talking about them or drawing them, you begin to gain a deeper understanding and a better grasp of them. Once you have some space between the thought, the fear, and the emotion, you can start to have some separation and make sense of them and develop new perspectives on them. This can help you to let go of old patterns of thinking and behavior that may have been holding you back.

CBT intervention: Face your fears

Avoidance only fuels anxiety, keeping you trapped in a cycle of intrusive thoughts and self-destructive behaviors. You have the power to break free from this pattern by courageously facing your fears head-on.

Anxiety can be likened to a gas that expands to fill whatever space you give it. It is fueled by fear and has the potential to consume your entire world if you allow it to. However, you have the power to contain it. You don't have to allow fear to dominate your thoughts, actions, and experiences. Instead, you have the power to establish firm boundaries and take control. When you become aware of its presence, make a deliberate choice to contain it. Place limits on the space it occupies in your life. For example, inform your anxiety that you are open to hearing all its concerns for the next 10 minutes, but beyond that, you are going to consciously dial it down.

So, how do you dial it down? Reach out to a friend and invest your energy in their struggles for a while. Take a leisurely walk while simultaneously contributing to your community by picking up litter. Nurture your creativity: engage in activities such as coloring in a book or playing a musical instrument. These actions empower you to reclaim control over your thoughts and emotions, diminishing the influence of fear. Remember, you are not helpless in the face of anxiety and fears.

Facing what scares you is hard, but facing fear is a crucial step in overcoming anxiety and taking control of your life. It may seem daunting. However, confronting the very things that makes you uncomfortable is the path to freedom. We will learn all those techniques in the following chapters, but first you need to identify what you are truly afraid of. Make a list of five things that scare the shit out of you. This is the first step.

Remember, it's normal to feel worse initially as you expose yourself to what scares you. However, by pushing through the temporary discomfort, you'll gradually weaken the hold anxiety has over you.

Time to do it!
List five things that scare the shit out of you.

Art Therapy exercise: Draw your inner monster

What is the one thing that you are most scared of? It could be anxiety, trauma, anger, resentment, grief, addiction, or the feeling of being unlovable or disliked by others. This exercise isn't about visualizing a specific person who may have caused you pain but rather focusing on the emotional residue left behind from a negative experience or relationship.

You are going to draw a monster that symbolizes this internal struggle and fear. Consider its color and shape—is it dark and menacing or perhaps more subdued? Does it have a prickly, soft, or slimy texture? Does it have claws, antennas, feathers, fabric, teeth, or any other defining features?

Explanation and discussion prompts

This monster represents your fears, anxiety, and feelings. It holds great significance. One important thing to remember is that the monster in your head always seems bigger and scarier than when you bring it out onto the paper. By externalizing it through your drawing, you create a tangible representation that can be contained within the boundaries of the piece of paper. This act of containment provides a sense of separation and perspective. When your fears and anxiety are confined to the paper, they do not feel so scary.

In addition, the monster is externalized, outside of your head, and not existing as a part of you. This separation allows you to establish a boundary between yourself and the monster in your mind. You create a visual reminder that these fears do not define you—they are separate entities that can be acknowledged and faced head-on.

Once you have completed your monster drawing, I encourage

you to take some time to ponder these thought-provoking questions as a way to further delve into your own experiences. Whether you prefer to engage in introspective journal writing or have a meaningful conversation or a coach, or a trusted friend, consider these questions as valuable starting points. Feel free to approach them in a way that feels most authentic to you, selecting the ones that truly resonate while skipping over any that may not quite align with your current journey.

1. Describe your monster—what color/shape is it?

2. If you were standing next to it, how big would you be?

3. Does it feel different looking at it now as opposed to when it is inside your head?

4. How did the process of creating this monster-drawing help you externalize and visualize your negative emotions?

5. What insights or realizations did you gain from observing your monster-drawing? Did anything surprise you?

6. How does interacting with your monster-drawing impact your relationship with those negative emotions? Does it provide any sense of distance or empowerment?

7. Reflecting on your experience of drawing your monster, how might this exercise influence your approach to managing and transforming negative emotions in your daily life?

8. What would you like to add/remove in order to change your monster?

Additional exercises, follow up, and next steps: Non-dominant hand conversation with the monster

To explore your inner relationship with fear, you are now going to talk to your monster. Start with a new blank sheet of paper. Take a black pen and hold it in your dominant hand. This pen represents the voice of your adult, rational self. The part of you that is logical and reasoned. Next, take the crayon or marker that you used to draw your monster and hold it in your non-dominant hand. This will symbolize your monster's voice, representing your fears and insecurities.

Begin this exercise by using your dominant hand to write down the question, "What do you want?" Next, use your non-dominant hand, and imagine this as your monster's voice, allowing it to express itself freely on the paper. In this process, you are giving your inner fear a chance to talk without any filters or judgments. Simply let the words flow naturally, allowing your fear to have a voice and express itself.

Avoid judging or filtering the responses. Instead, let the words flow naturally onto the paper, allowing your fear to have a voice. Engage in a dialogue between the two voices on the paper. Explore the relationship between your adult rational self and your fear. Ideally ending in understanding each other and finding a potential resolution.

You will know when you are nearing the end of the dialogue. You will have to steer the conversation into a place where you are empowered and yet empathetic toward your monster. Try using a phrase such as "I hear you and I appreciate you." Then add, "But you will no longer control me."

I believe that our fears are akin to a small child trying to get our attention. They will continue to get louder and louder the more we ignore them. Your fear likes to yell and scream. However, just like a child who is prone to tantrums, if you give them your attention, let them talk, and then set boundaries with love, you will appease the fear while staying in control.

1. Start by asking the monster, "What do you want?"

2. Write at least a full page.

3. End by telling it something such as "I appreciate you" or "I hear/see you" or "Thank you." Then add, "But you will no longer control me."

My client, Brad, was a people pleaser. He'd spent years struggling with being able to stand up for himself in varied situations—meetings at work, relationships with family and friends, and even in grocery store lines. As a child he'd been told that he wasn't good enough by his father, and in turn, Brad had met with failure in school and in the sports his father had made him participate in. He'd grown into an adult who was blindingly afraid of criticism but infuriated with himself for caring about what others thought of him. He felt worthless, like a nobody, afraid to make a change, to speak out. When directed to draw his monster he created a blue dragon. It was angry.

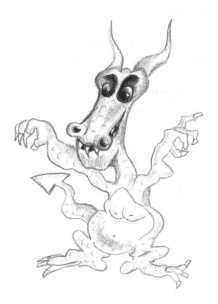

With a black pen firmly held in his dominant hand, symbolizing his rational self, and a blue pencil grasped in his non-dominant hand, embodying his inner angry monster, his conversation unfolded as follows:

Brad (dominant hand): What do you want?

Dragon (non-dominant hand): I want control! I want you to believe that you are worthless.

Brad (dominant hand): I refuse to let you define my worth.

Dragon (non-dominant hand): You're nothing! You've failed before, and you'll fail again!

Brad (dominant hand): I acknowledge my past struggles, but they don't define me.

Dragon (non-dominant hand): You're delusional. You're going to fail at everything.

Brad (dominant hand): I am more than my fuck-ups.

Dragon (non-dominant hand): You're just fooling yourself. You'll never be good enough.

Brad (dominant hand): I choose not to believe your lies. I have the power to see my own worth.

Dragon (non-dominant hand): Fine, whatever! You're going to do what you are going to do.

Brad (dominant hand): Thank you for acknowledging that. I am stronger than you.

Dragon (non-dominant hand): I am just trying to protect you from getting hurt. You don't even appreciate me.

Brad (dominant hand): I see you and I hear you. Thank you for watching out for me, but I got this!

As Brad finished the conversation, he looked at the artwork before him and the dialogue between his rational self and the dragon's voice. It stood as a testament to his desired resilience and determination. Brad knew that by confronting his fears, he could reclaim his power. This exercise showed Brad that he could be in control of his own worth and forge a path of self-acceptance and empowerment. It all begins with a willingness to talk to the parts of ourselves that try to derail us—for whatever reason—and know that fears do not define us.

What do you want?
I want control! I want you to believe you are worthless.
I refuse to let you define my worth.
You're nothing! You've failed before, and you'll fail again!
I acknowledge my past struggles, but they don't define me.
You're delusional. You're going fail at everything.
I am more than my F-ups.
You're just fooling. You're going to fail at everything.
I choose not to believe your lies. I have the power
to see my own worth.
Fine, whatever! You're going to what you are going to do.
Thank you for acknowledging that I am stronger than
you. I am just trying to protect you from getting hurt.
You don't even appreciate me.
I see you and I hear you. Thank you for
watching out for me, but I got this!

The conversation between you and your inner monster represents your internal struggle with self-doubt and negative self-talk. This Art Therapy exercise acknowledges the presence of your inner critic and confronts its negative influence. Through your dominant hand, your rational self, you strive for growth and success. Your non-dominant hand, representing your inner monster, embodies all those insecurities and negative thoughts that hold you back. The conversation is an opportunity to confront self-doubt and choose a more empowering mindset. Don't let your inner monster define who you are; instead, give the monster the opportunity to speak while you listen.

It is beneficial to express gratitude toward the monster or extend love and compassion to it. This approach establishes a foundation for integrating the different aspects of your personality, leading to a more unified and harmonious self. If your conversation did not conclude with a sense of empowerment and self-confidence, persist in the dialogue until you can hear yourself say: "I am strong and I recognize that I have choices" or "Hey monster, I choose not to listen to you anymore."

Below are some further questions to help you explore the dialogue with your monster:

- What came up for you?

- In what ways was it easy/ difficult?

- Were you surprised by anything that you wrote?

- What did you feel at the beginning of the writing? And by the end?

"*When you can make the unconscious conscious, that can dissipate the emotional charge.*" Your experience with the artwork and the internal dialogue you had with the monster is a powerful example of this. You see, when these fears hide in the shadows of your mind, they can have this commanding, negative impact on your emotions and actions. But by bringing them into the light of consciousness and actively dealing with them, you started to weaken their hold on you.

NOTES FOR THERAPISTS

Begin your third session with the above quotation and the goal of externalizing fear. Then review the homework previously assigned by asking your client what new ANTs (automatic negative thoughts) came up for them and what are the PANTs (present affirming nurturing thoughts) that they used to replace them? Lead your client through the "Face your fear" CBT exercise followed by a discussion. Then dedicate at least 15 minutes to having your client drawing their monster.

Given that you and your client have already completed the CBT exercise and the monster drawing during your 50-minute session, there may not be sufficient time to undertake the non-dominant hand conversation in this session. This additional Art Therapy exercise is most effective when assigned as homework. It's crucial to clearly explain the instructions to your client and ensure they comprehend the process, including how to initiate and conclude the conversation.

CHAPTER FOUR

Fourth Module:
Stay in the Present Moment and Change Your Perspective

Naomi Judd was an American singer, songwriter, and actress, who is said to have made an astute observation about the profound link between our mental and physical well-being: *"Your body hears everything your mind says."*[5] It underscores the significance of being mindful of our thoughts and emotions in nurturing both our mental and physical health. We need to be mindful of our self-talk, as our body reacts to it. Continuously telling ourselves we're tired or anxious will make our body feel that way. Conversely, affirming our strength, health, and gratitude will shape how we perceive the world and how our body responds. Despite her evident awareness of this connection between self-talk and well-being, it's a tragic reality that Naomi herself succumbed to the weight of those negative inner voices, ultimately leading to taking her own life by suicide. This poignant example illustrates that even when we are cognizant of what is beneficial for us, we may not always do the right thing—highlighting the complex and often challenging nature of our inner struggles.

Goal: Learning to see another perspective

Today, you have three important goals.

First, I encourage you to recognize that feelings, even when uncomfortable, are not harmful. They're simply emotions, and you can acquire the ability to tolerate them without resorting to self-destructive behaviors to escape them.

Second, it's crucial to understand that there is often more than one perspective to consider when dealing with a feeling or a situation.

Lastly, our third goal is to establish a connection between emotions and the physical sensations in the body. We'll delve into identifying where in the body you experience these emotions.

During my time facilitating Art Therapy groups at drug treatment centers in Los Angeles, I encountered numerous instances where participants would become frustrated with the art process and feel the urge to give up or leave the group. In those moments, I would remind them that in the past, whenever they faced uncomfortable feelings like frustration, their go-to response was to numb those emotions with substances such as alcohol or drugs. However, now, in the journey of recovery, it was essential for them to learn a different approach—to learn to tolerate those challenging emotions head-on.

The frustration they experienced while creating imperfect art became a pivotal opportunity for growth. It was a time where they could sit in that feeling without resorting to substances, anger, shame, or avoidance. By staying present in that discomfort and resisting the old, unproductive coping mechanisms, they were actively practicing emotional resilience and fostering personal transformation.

In those Art Therapy sessions, participants gradually learned to celebrate progress over perfection and build a healthy relationship with their emotions. Through art, they discovered a safe space for self-expression, self-reflection, and the exploration of their inner landscape.

As they persevered through the frustrating moments, they began to witness their own resilience and capacity for growth. The art became a tangible symbol of their journey, a testament to their willingness to face discomfort and cultivate healthier coping strategies.

CBT intervention: Learning to see the good in the bad

In every situation, there are invariably elements that encompass both positive and negative aspects. Embracing the positive doesn't demand dismissing the negative; rather, it involves the act of uncovering those subtle glimpses of brightness within the darkest of circumstances. This shift in perspective can have a profound impact, ultimately lifting your mood and fostering resilience.

For this exercise, I'd like you to identify a challenging situation you've faced in your life, and then uncover a positive outcome or experience that arose from it. In your journal, complete the sentence: "If it weren't for [the challenging situation], I would have never [positive outcome or experience]."

This exercise encourages you to reframe adversity and discover the hidden silver linings in your life's journey.

> For example, my client, Graham, came to me after he was unexpectedly laid off from work. He was devastated, scared, and feeling worthless. When he received the unexpected news of his layoff, it initially struck him as disheartening. However, little did he know that this setback would ignite the fire within him to pursue his entrepreneurial aspirations.
>
> Graham wrote, "If it weren't for being laid off from work, I would never have started my own business."
>
> Losing his job turned out to be the catalyst Graham needed. It provided him with the motivation to transform his dreams into reality. He channeled his time, energy, and expertise, which he'd honed over years of professional experience, into developing his own business concept.

In this way, even a difficult situation like a job loss can lead to unexpected and positive outcomes, showcasing the power of finding the positive amid adversity.

What are some of your silver linings? Write them out now.

Art Therapy exercise: Feeling Poem and Drawing

This Art Therapy exercise begins with a writing prompt. Don't fret about not being a skilled poet or adhering to rhyming schemes. Don't even worry about spelling things correctly or sticking to punctuation rules. The task is to create a poem following a specific structure.

First, I ask my client to name the uncomfortable feeling that they have been focused on during the past few sessions. It could be anxiety, anger, disappointment, loss, frustration, or any other emotion. Next, they choose a color that represents that particular feeling. There are two parts to the poem; both will be written with this one color.

My client Judy opted for the word "anxiety" and the color green. Example: Judy's poem (part 1):

Anxiety is green
Anxiety tastes like vinegar
Anxiety smells like pickles
Anxiety sounds like a slamming door
Anxiety looks like mold
Anxiety feels like gooey mud at the bottom of a lake
Anxiety comes from my thoughts

Your turn. Use this simple format as your guide.

⊛ FEELING POEM (PART 1)

. . . . is . . . .
My feeling   *Color*

. . . . tastes like . . . .
My feeling

. . . . smells like . . . .
My feeling

. . . . sounds like . . . .
My feeling

. . . . looks like . . . .
My feeling

. . . . feels like . . . .
My feeling

. . . . comes from . . . .
My feeling

The second part of the poem explores the polar opposite of the original feeling. I ask my clients to choose a word that is in contrast to their original feeling. I tell them to embrace this new feeling as they craft the same poem, but they must use the same color as before—no switching allowed.

Judy chose "calm" as the opposite feeling to "anxiety" and proceeded with her green marker for the second part of the poem. She wrote:

> Calm is green
> Calm tastes like green tea ice cream
> Calm smells like fresh cut grass
> Calm sounds like a river flowing by
> Calm looks like trees swaying in the breeze
> Calm feels like my cat's soft, warm fur
> Calm comes from my thoughts

Your turn (part 2)—use your original color and the same format as your guide.

⊕ FEELING POEM (PART 2)

. . . . .is . . . .
My opposite feeling   *Same color*

. . . . .tastes like . . . .
My opposite feeling

. . . . .smells like. . . . .
My opposite feeling

. . . . .sounds like . . . .
My opposite feeling

. . . . .looks like. . . . .
My opposite feeling

. . . . .feels like . . . .
My opposite feeling

. . . . .comes from . . . .
My opposite feeling

After finishing both parts of the poem, set the poem aside and go to the next blank page in your journal, or grab a blank sheet of white paper. You can draw anything you want on this paper—using any colors. No limits or specific instructions. I call this a "free drawing." There are no restrictions in this artistic endeavor. Let your creativity take over and enjoy the process of drawing!

Following her Feeling Poem, Judy drew a black cat curled under a huge green dripping ice cream cone.

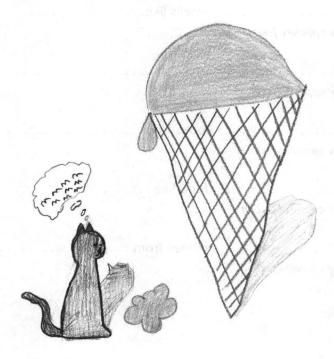

Explanation and discussion prompts

By using one color for both the uncomfortable feeling and the opposite feeling, I encourage my clients to recognize and embrace the interconnectedness of their emotions. I have found that it highlights the concept of positive and negative emotions co-existing within the same person, even at the same time. They are not mutually exclusive.

In addition, instructing my clients to stick with a single color provides them the opportunity to explore and redefine the associations and meanings they attach to that color. They become aware that the color itself is neutral, and it is their labeling that gives it emotional meaning.

I have witnessed my clients recognizing that they have the power to change the associations they attribute to the color. It illustrates their ability to transform their perspective on the meaning they give to other things that they may have identified as a "trigger."

I often come across people who say, "I can't do XYZ because it triggers me." Many people avoid specific things due to the negative memories associated with them. I want them to stop avoiding what is hard. For many individuals, shying away from frightening or uncomfortable situations isn't conducive to their well-being. In fact, it's my therapeutic recommendation to confront those challenges head-on, even when they feel daunting and scary. I never suggest anything I wouldn't do myself. Whether it's skiing after a decade of being off the slopes or having a tough conversation with a loved one, I often find myself admitting, "This really scares me, but that won't stop me from doing it."

One of my clients, Aaron, was undergoing treatment for heroin addiction. He expressed discomfort when I suggested using aluminum foil in an art project. He firmly stated, "I can't use aluminum foil because it triggers me." (Aluminum foil is commonly used in the inhalation method of consuming heroin.)

In response, I reminded Aaron that there was a time in his life, before he started using heroin, when aluminum foil had no negative associations for him. I pointed out that he had assigned meaning to that household item based on his past behavior.

I urged him to engage in the art project using aluminum foil and to confront his discomfort head-on. By doing so, he could begin creating new experiences and memories.

Over time, as Aaron embraced the challenge and persisted in using aluminum foil, it gradually transformed from being a triggering item to a neutral one. This shift in perception allowed him to detach the negative associations he had attributed to it and approach it without distress.

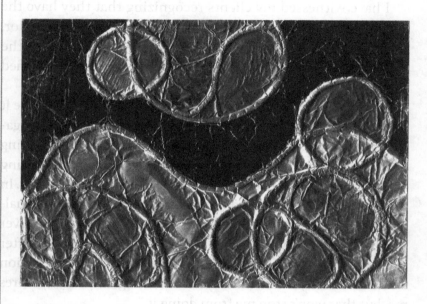

Guiding Aaron to confront his discomfort and reframe his relationship with aluminum foil helped him to break free from the limitations imposed by his past experiences. This process enabled him to create new, positive associations and expand his capacity for personal growth and healing.

That is why I encourage my clients to stick with the same color for both the negative and positive feelings, even when they may be inclined to choose a different color. It's important to challenge their usual patterns and comfort zones because true change and growth happen outside of those familiar spaces.

It is useful to reflect on your experience of writing the poem and creating the drawing. These thought-provoking prompts can be effective tools in facilitating a meaningful and transformative therapeutic journey.

1. How did writing this poem help you in exploring and expressing your experience of your two feelings?

2. How do the sensory descriptions (taste, smell, sound, look, and feel) in your poem enhance your understanding of your two feelings?

3. Did any specific emotions or memories arise for you?

4. In what ways do you think your perception might have shifted or deepened through the process of writing this poem?

5. How might you apply the insights gained from this poem to better understand and manage your own yucky feelings, and cultivate a sense of mental wellness in your life?

6. How did the sensory descriptions in the poem deepen your awareness of the physical sensations associated with anxiety and calm within your own body?

7. You probably wanted to switch colors for the second part of the poem; why do you think you were asked to keep the same color?

8. Tell me about your drawing.

   a. Does it relate to the poem in any way?

   b. Did you use the original color? Did you choose to leave it out?

Additional exercises, follow up, and next steps: Rewrite the Feeling Poem (with a different feeling!)

This is fairly simple—I encourage you to revisit this exercise of creating a poem and drawing, but this time, pick a different word to begin with. This will allow you to explore another emotion that you have been struggling with. This can offer you a new viewpoint. It's akin to examining your emotions from a different angle, potentially providing you with fresh insights into your fears and motivations.

For example, if you initially used the word "fear" for your poem, consider beginning with the word "disappointed" this time around. Be sure to select a color that accurately symbolizes "disappointed." Let's see where this new starting point leads you. Don't forget to follow up your poem with a drawing of anything you feel like drawing.

"Your body hears everything your mind says" emphasizes that our mental state, thoughts, and emotions are not isolated from our physical bodies. Rather, through your Feeling Poem, you engaged all five of your senses, immersing yourself in the sensation of discomfort on various levels. It's a crucial aspect of this journey to develop the capacity to withstand discomfort for a brief period without resorting to self-destructive behavior. However, the latter part of the poem enabled you to immerse yourself in positive emotions through all your senses, and I'm willing to bet your body truly responded to that uplifting experience. It's intentional that I had you conclude your poem with the positive feeling because I aim for those to be the last words your mind and body embrace. This way, you are left with those uplifting emotions.

NOTES FOR THERAPISTS
When your client returns for the fourth session, start by introducing Naomi Judd's quotation and outlining the session's objectives. Following this, request that they read their non-dominant hand conversation aloud and encourage them to share their experience with the exercise.

However, if your client couldn't complete the non-dominant hand conversation as homework, consider dedicating the beginning of the session to this exercise, as it is a vital component of this program.

Guide your client through the "Learning to see the good in the bad" CBT exercise and follow that up with a discussion. Suggest that your client take brief notes for future reference, or if they prefer, they can document their thoughts in their journal, even though this option may consume more session time. Additionally, make sure both the Feeling Poem and Drawing exercise are completed within the session.

For homework, encourage your client to explore the Feeling Poem exercise with a different emotion, and discuss during the next session. Assigning homework to your client serves the purpose of maintaining the therapeutic process between sessions.

Clients often find verbal and visual examples of the Feeling Poem exercises particularly valuable. Don't hesitate to use the case studies provided in this book or incorporate examples from your own professional background. Or, if you are feeling brave, share your own Feeling Poems.

CHAPTER FIVE

Fifth Module:
Separate Physical Symptoms, Thoughts, and Behaviors

David Duchovny is an American actor and director who often portrays dark, anxious characters. In several interviews he has openly discussed his own struggles with addiction and other mental health issues, one time stating, *"Anxiety is part of creativity: the need to get something out, to get rid of something, or get in touch with something deep within."*[6] This quotation illustrates that by tapping into our innermost thoughts and feelings, we can find inspiration and meaning in our lives, and use our creativity to express ourselves in new and profound ways.

Anxiety can arise from a variety of sources, such as uncertainty, fear, or insecurity. These feelings can create a sense of urgency in individuals, prompting them to take action and find solutions to the challenges they face. In the creative process, this sense of urgency can manifest itself as a need to express oneself through art, writing, music, or other creative outlets.

Goal: Separating physical symptoms from thoughts and behaviors

Circling back to Erin, I'd like to share something she discovered as she progressed through the Creative Cognitive Therapy method. She said, "I feel like the drawings are becoming easier because I know what to expect, and I've done them several times." She and I discussed how, in general, high-functioning adults often dislike doing things for the first time because it feels uncomfortable when they don't yet have the skills. We tend to prefer doing things we're already good at. However, there's a simple truth: Anything we do repeatedly becomes easier. In other words, the more we repeat a behavior, understand it, and develop the necessary skills, the easier it becomes. Easy isn't something that's given; it's something we achieve through practice and effort.

With that said, I want to commend you for sticking with this process, no matter how easy or frustrating it may be. Keep pushing through; you're on the right track.

This module is designed with two primary objectives in mind. The first goal focuses on separating your physical symptoms from your thoughts. By recognizing that physical sensations are distinct from thoughts and behaviors, you can disentangle the various elements contributing to your distress. This separation empowers you to better comprehend the impact of your thoughts and behaviors on your emotional well-being. It enables you to intervene and make positive changes in your thought patterns and behaviors, ultimately reducing the intensity and duration of distressing symptoms.

The second objective is all about giving you the tools to regain control when things feel overwhelming. It's about helping you to effectively recognize strategies that can break those harmful patterns and replace them with behaviors that boost your overall well-being. In essence, it provides you with a clear plan of action.

CBT intervention: Would you say that to a child?

We all have those automatic negative thoughts (ANTs) that infiltrate our brain. Imagine what damage would be done if you said those things to a child. Our inner critic says things that we would (hopefully!) never say to a child such as "you're too fat" or "you'll never be good enough." We find it easier to be empathetic and compassionate toward others, especially children, but we can be overly critical and harsh toward ourselves. We often personalize our mistakes and failures, viewing them as reflections of our worth, while being more forgiving and understanding when children make mistakes, even reframing those mistakes as learning opportunities.

Negative self-talk can be learned from our upbringing and environment, especially if criticism was prevalent. Recognizing this is crucial to challenge and transform negative self-talk. By telling yourself the same things you would say to encourage a child, you can cultivate self-compassion, gradually shifting the inner dialogue toward a healthier and more nurturing mindset.

Think about the kind of messages that would empower, encourage, and let a child know they are loved. Write down at least five statements of love and encouragement. Now, imagine saying these very same things to yourself, using your own name when addressing yourself. There is power in saying your own name. Make it a daily practice to speak these affirmations to yourself for the next week:

For instance, I would say:

"You have the power to overcome challenges, Pamela."

"Pamela, you are strong and capable."

"Pamela, you are loved and cherished just as you are."

Art Therapy exercise: Anxiety timeline

This next Art Therapy exercise may seem complex. However, I've taken great care to break it down into 10 simple steps that effectively guide you through the process. Prior to embarking on this exercise, bear with me while we go through some brief psychoeducation emphasizing the significance of distinguishing between thoughts and physical sensations.

It's common for people to blend their physical sensations with their thoughts, treating them as a single entity. However, it is tremendously beneficial to separate these two aspects in order to comprehend how seemingly simple anxiety can swiftly escalate into intense panic. To illustrate this, let's consider the example of driving. If a car cuts me off in traffic, my body immediately reacts with a surge of adrenaline. This results in a racing heart, shallow breaths, and a hot, tingling sensation. We can label these physical sensations as "first fear."[7] It's important to note that our body has the ability to self-regulate, and these symptoms will naturally decrease and dissipate within a few minutes.

Unfortunately, it is our thoughts about these physical sensations that escalate our anxiety further. We may find ourselves thinking: "My heart is racing; I must be having a heart attack" or "I can't breathe; I'm going to faint." These thoughts can be termed "second fear."[8] By recognizing these two elements as separate entities, we can understand that the physiological reaction is a normal response. This realization allows us to interrupt catastrophic thoughts before they worsen the situation.

This Art Therapy exercise involves constructing a timeline that illustrates the process, starting with the physical sensations, then adding the catastrophic thoughts, and identifying opportunities for cognitive and behavioral changes that can interrupt this timeline. Refer to the examples below. These will be helpful. Now, let's explore the steps involved in this Art Therapy exercise:

1. Think about the times when your fear or anxiety felt overwhelming.

2. Identify the physical sensations experienced during those moments and represent each sensation using a different shape and color. These are the "first fear" sensations.

   a. Example: shallow breathing = light blue waves.

   b. Example: racing heart = a red heart.

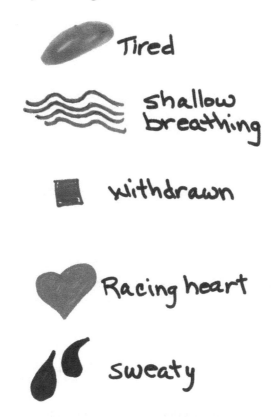

Step 2: Example of symbols and shapes to represent your physical/somatic reactions when you are overwhelmed

Key: Tired = brown blob, shallow breathing = purple wavy lines, withdrawn = green square, racing heart = red heart, sweaty = blue water drops
You can choose your own shapes and colors

3. On a separate piece of paper, create a scale ranging from 0 to 10 to represent the intensity of the feeling.

   a. Start at the lower left-hand side of a piece of paper and write the numbers 0 through 10.

   b. Zero equals no symptoms and 10 is the most extreme symptoms.

10
9
8
7
6
5
4
3
2
1
0

Step 3: Example of the anxiety scale
Write numbers from bottom to top on the left side of the paper

4. Draw a line that represents the progression of your feeling.

   a. How quickly does that feeling intensify?

   b. How long does it remain elevated at an uncomfortable level?

   c. How long does it take to come back to neutral?

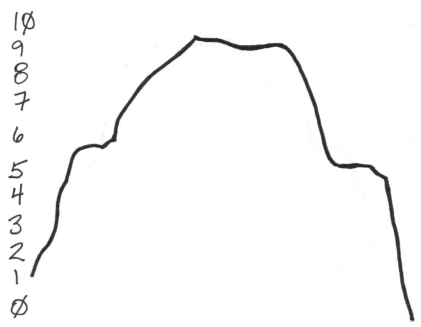

Step 4: Example of the anxiety scale with timeline moving
left to right (this often looks like a mountain)
*Draw a line that represents the progression of your
panic attack (any uncomfortable feeling)*

5. Plot the physical sensations along the timeline to indicate when they occur.

   a. Use the colored shapes from step 2.

   b. Put all these colored shapes below the timeline.

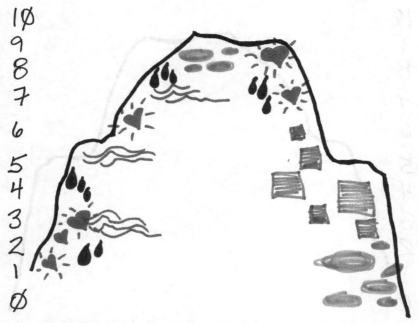

Step 5: Example of the physical sensations occurring along the timeline
Note that all these colored shapes are below the timeline

6. Write down your Automatic Negative Thoughts (ANTs) on the timeline where they emerge.

   a. This is "second fear."

   b. Example: at level 3, with a racing heart, the ANT may be "I am having a heart attack."

   c. Example: at level 7, when feeling sweaty, the ANT may be "I am so embarrassed."

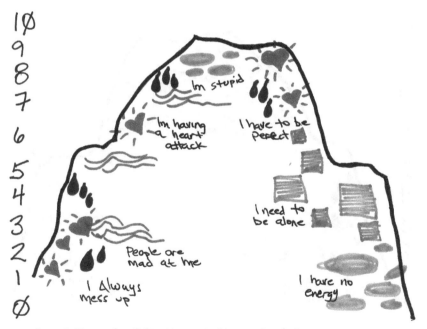

Step 6: Example of the ANTs on the timeline where they emerge

7. Rip or cut strips of paper to cover up the ANTs.

8. Replace the ANTs with Present and Affirming Nurturing Thoughts (PANTs) by writing new statements on those strips of paper and taping them on top of, or next to, each old statement.

    a. This is cognitive restructuring.

    b. Example: "I am having a heart attack" is changed to "My heart is beating."

    c. Example: "I am so embarrassed" is changed to "I am confident."

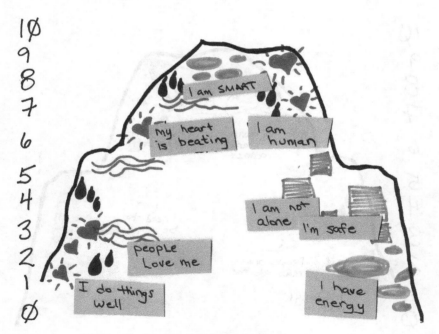

Steps 7 and 8: Example of the PANTs written on strips of paper and taped on top of the ANTs

9. Use simple shapes and colors to represent healthy behaviors.

   a. Example: deep breathing = dark blue cloud.

   b. Example: go outside = orange arrow.

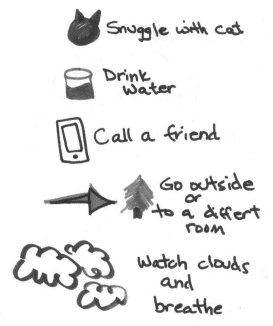

Step 9: Example of shapes and colors to represent new healthy behaviors
*Key: Snuggle with cat = brown cat, drink water = purple glass of water, call a friend =
black mobile phone, go outside = orange arrow, watch clouds and breathe = blue clouds*
Plot those healthy behaviors along the timeline

c. This is behavioral intervention.

10. Plot all these new healthy behaviors, represented by colored shapes, above the line. Use this visual cue to remind yourself when to incorporate these new behaviors during stressful times.

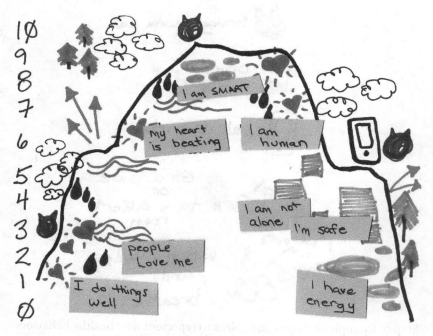

Step 10: Example of healthy behaviors along the timeline

Explanation and discussion prompts

I want to acknowledge the numerous steps involved in the Art Therapy exercise—and you have successfully completed them all! Let's take a moment to appreciate everything you accomplished. You were able to distinguish your physical sensations from the thoughts that tend to catastrophize the future. This separation allows you to slow down the process and challenge those thoughts by focusing on the present moment. It's a powerful tool for regaining control over your thinking patterns.

Furthermore, you have identified healthy behaviors that you can adopt to provide support for yourself during difficult times. By pinpointing the precise moments in your timeline where these behaviors would be most beneficial, you have created a clear roadmap for taking positive steps forward.

When you look at the entire exercise, you'll notice that it has a clear beginning, middle, and end. This is a good reminder that even when the feelings become overwhelming, they eventually diminish and/or end. By consistently practicing cognitive restructuring and implementing behavioral changes, you'll witness a reduction in the intensity and frequency of these episodes over time.

I want to emphasize that your dedication to this process and your commitment to regularly implementing these strategies will lead to positive results. The tools you've acquired will support your journey as we continue toward greater emotional well-being.

1. What else do you notice when you look at your completed timeline?

2. What have you learned from this exercise?

3. How/when can you use this?

4. Are there any other healthy behaviors that you can add to your timeline?

Additional exercises, follow up, and next steps

There are two different assignments.

1. Add any new and additional healthy behaviors to the time-line (if needed), such as stretching, creating a gratitude list (see next chapter), or doing something creative.

2. Redraw: What you are carrying/holding (2nd time). Add things you are releasing/letting go of.

Remember the Art Therapy exercise you did in Session 2, where you drew yourself holding all your automatic negative thoughts (ANTs)? Well, it's time to revisit that. I want you to just think about all the ANTs that you are still carrying around. Unfortunately, we never get rid of all of them, but maybe at this point you have released or changed some of those. You may also have new or additional ANTs that you have become aware of during the last few sessions.

Without going back and looking at your original drawing, you are going to again draw yourself holding all those burdens. As a reminder, here are the directions again:

1. Begin by drawing a person to represent yourself. This can be as simple as a stick person or more detailed. You can choose any pose or position that feels authentic to you. It does not have to be too complicated.

2. Imagine yourself holding or carrying several objects (these represent your many ANTs). Decide how you are carrying the objects. It could be in your hands, on your head, on your back, on your shoulders, or even with your feet. The placement could reflect the weight or impact of your ANTs.

3. This is the additional step: If you feel that you have started to release some of those negative thoughts, draw yourself letting go of those objects. That could look like you are tossing some away, releasing some into the sky, or letting them drop to the ground.

4. Once you are completely done with this drawing, you can take out the original drawing from Session 2 and compare and contrast them.

ERIN'S STORY

After completing her second drawing and comparing it to the first, Erin made some insightful observations. In the second rendition of the "What you are carrying/holding" exercise, she redrew the same objects but noticed a significant change. Now, only half of the objects floated around her, while she held onto four of them. When discussing this transformation, Erin remarked, "These are the things I feel like I am getting a hold of." In addition, she pointed out that the figure in the initial drawing was leaning to the left, creating a sense of instability. Erin was surprised to see that in the second drawing she had depicted the figure standing upright with a smile, describing it as feeling more grounded and stable.

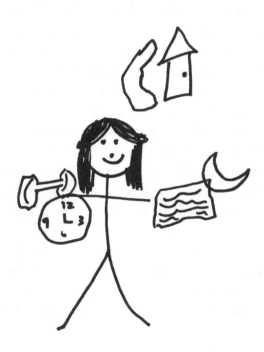

As you reach the conclusion of this module, it's important to understand that anxieties and fears are natural emotions that you'll never completely eliminate. They have a purpose in our lives. Keep in mind the words of wisdom: Anxiety is an integral part of creativity. It's the drive to express, release, or connect with something deep within. Use it as your spark of creativity. Instead of trying to suppress it, learn to listen to these feelings and acknowledge them, but don't let them take over and control your life.

NOTES FOR THERAPISTS

Start the fifth session by introducing the quotation from Duchovny and outlining the goals for the session. Take a few minutes to revisit the "Feeling Poem" assignment, which your client worked on as homework. Encourage your client to share their poem by reading it out loud and discuss any thoughts or feelings that arose during this process.

Next, guide your client through the "Would you say that to a child?" CBT exercise. Following the exercise, engage in a comprehensive discussion to explore their insights. Suggest that they take any notes to refer back to later.

Ensure that they complete all the steps of the "Anxiety timeline" exercise during this session.

For homework, assign two tasks. First, ask your client to update their timeline with any new strategies or thoughts that may emerge during the week. This ongoing process keeps them actively engaged in fostering positive changes and helps them become more aware of negative thoughts until your next session.

The second homework assignment involves revisiting and redrawing the "What you are carrying/holding" picture from the second module. Encourage your client to consider adding any additional negative thoughts they might be holding onto and prompt them to reflect on whether they are ready to let go of these thoughts. They should depict themselves releasing these negative thoughts in their drawing, whether by tossing them away, releasing them into the sky, or letting them gently fall to the ground. Stress that they should rely on their memory for this task, rather than revisiting the original drawing, to highlight the differences between memory and reality.

You can provide these homework instructions in writing for your client to take home as a reminder or go over them in detail during the session's conclusion to ensure they fully understand and can effectively complete the assignments.

Sixth Module:
Consciously Switch to a Gratitude Mind

Philosopher, teacher, and author Eckhart Tolle suggested that we should embrace whatever is happening to us right now. He said: *"Whatever the present moment contains, accept it as if you had chosen it. Always work with it, not against it. Make it your friend and ally, not your enemy. This will miraculously transform your whole life."*[9] By accepting the present moment, we can avoid creating unnecessary stress and tension in our lives. Instead of constantly trying to change or control the present, we can focus on making the most of the situation and finding ways to grow and learn from it.

Tolle's spiritual journey started at 29 years of age when he was feeling particularly overwhelmed and hopeless. He contemplated suicide. Perhaps it was staring down at his own mortality that drew him inward. He felt an intense stillness inside himself and his sense of "self" dissolved as he became aware of a presence or consciousness that was beyond his individual identity. His perception of the world was, from that time on, altered.

Goals: Gaining control of your perspective

Being in control of our perspective is crucial for mental wellness because it shapes how we perceive and interpret the world around us. It influences our thoughts, emotions, and behaviors, ultimately impacting our overall well-being.

You may think there is only one possible reality for your life, and you are forced to accept whatever happens to you. But there are many potentialities depending on where you are and what you are focused on.

The other day my dear friend Patrick and I were standing in front of a sculpture in an art gallery. As we talked about our interpretations, we discovered that we were viewing the same sculpture from different perspectives.

Patrick, an architect, approached the sculpture from a structural perspective. Being trained in understanding forms and spatial relationships, Patrick saw the sleek, geometric lines and polished surfaces as representing contemporary skyscrapers and urban landscapes. For him, the sculpture evoked feelings of efficiency, precision, and the power of human creativity.

On the other hand, as an art therapist, I approached the sculpture from an emotional and psychological perspective. I saw the sculpture as a portrayal of the human psyche and inner struggles. The tangled and intertwined metal elements resonated with me. It evoked feelings of vulnerability, inner turmoil, and the potential for growth and transformation.

It's not just about what we have been taught that influences our perspective. It is also about what meaning we assign to any given situation. For example, below are two very different interpretations of the exact same circumstances:

Perspective 1: What a day I had. I was stuck in traffic for hours, rushing between three different jobs. After a long arduous day, dinner with my friends turned into a frustrating experience. The waiter was complaining about the staff, the service was slow, and our orders were incorrect. It felt like everything went wrong today!

Perspective 2: What a day I had! I had the opportunity to drive along the Pacific Coast Highway, enjoying the breathtaking views and the refreshing ocean breeze. Witnessing a kite-boarder in action added an extra touch of excitement to my day. I'm grateful to have three jobs that I can easily commute to. After work, I met up with my friends for dinner, and it turned into a hilarious and memorable experience. Our waiter had a great sense of humor, joking about his own scatterbrain mishaps. We spent hours laughing and sharing stories. Even when I received the wrong food, it turned out to be a pleasant surprise and even better than what I had originally ordered. What a day: everything turned out better than I could have planned!

These two perspectives demonstrate how different interpretations can arise from the same set of events. They emphasize the power of focusing on positive aspects even when faced with challenges. This mindset shift, which I refer to as "gratitude mind," empowers us to intentionally seek out things to be grateful for, even in undesirable circumstances. It reminds us that by consciously choosing a brighter perspective, we can uncover the silver linings. This practice enables us to make the most out of every situation, fostering resilience, and enhancing our overall well-being.

Sometimes it can be very difficult to see another perspective, because we are so caught up in the frustration of the moment. To make it easier, there are three steps that are helpful in changing your perspective. And these three steps are your three goals for this module.

Goal 1: Accept your current circumstance as it is. This is key. Many times, we have specific expectations about how things should unfold, and when they deviate from that script, frustration sets in. While it's natural to feel disappointed, dwelling on the fact that things didn't go as planned is a drain on your energy. It's more productive to acknowledge the new situation you're in. This way, you can better analyze it, find solutions, and take steps to progress forward.

Goal 2: Stay in the present moment. Staying in the now is crucial for our emotional well-being. Jumping into the future and imagining the worst-case scenarios is a sure-fire way to negatively impact our mood. Alternatively, keeping your focus on what's happening right now can make you feel more stable and peaceful. It stops you from getting caught up in worrying about what might go wrong in the future (more about this concept in the next section).

Goal 3: Consciously switch to "gratitude mind." When life throws you a curveball, one of the best things you can do is seek out moments of gratitude. It won't alter the situation, but it will significantly brighten your outlook. Challenge yourself with statements like, "Yes, this unfortunate event just occurred, but at least..." and find three aspects to be thankful for. I understand that this is never easy. It requires a lot of practice. However, when you can master a "gratitude mindset," you'll be amazed at the results.

CBT intervention: Put your crystal ball away

A significant aspect of anxiety revolves around predicting catastrophic outcomes, but the truth is, these predictions are often highly inaccurate. You *cannot* predict the future. It's time to set aside the crystal ball and open yourself up to the possibility that there are numerous potential outcomes to any given situation. Remember, your imagination has the capacity to envision a multitude of potential positive *and* adverse results.

Here is your challenge: Think about one current worry and write out different ways it *could* turn out (good, bad, and neutral).

My client, Derick, had been practicing staying present for several weeks when he was summoned into his boss's office. His heart started racing. His mind filled with dread as he assumed the worst. Thoughts of being fired fueled his anxiety. However, he reminded himself that he did not have a crystal ball and he could not see the future. He told himself that there were many possibilities beyond his initial fear. Rather than succumbing to catastrophic thinking, Derick considered alternative outcomes that could possibly await him in that pivotal meeting. Below is Derick's list of the eight different ways that his meeting with his boss could go:

- Derick is fired.

- Derick is told he is on probation for an error that he made.

- Derick's boss wants to discuss a minor issue or concern that can be resolved through a constructive conversation.

- Derick is assigned a new project or responsibility that aligns with his skills and interests.

- Derick is recognized for his exceptional performance and is given a promotion or a raise.

- Derick receives positive feedback on his recent work and is praised for his contributions to the team.

- Derick and his family are invited to join his boss on a vacation weekend to their cabin by the lake.

- His boss asks Derick for his opinion regarding getting a dog (this one made Derick smile).

Gratitude is an essential part of reducing anxiety and developing a healthier mindset. By practicing gratitude, you train your mind to appreciate the good things, no matter how small, which helps to counterbalance the negative bias that often fuels anxiety. This shift in perspective allows you to cultivate a sense of contentment, resilience, and perspective. Additionally, gratitude encourages you to acknowledge and appreciate the present moment, grounding you in the here and now, rather than ruminating on past regrets or future uncertainties.

It is also important to be grateful for any loss or pain because it allows you to find meaning and growth even in the midst of challenging experiences. Having gratitude for our challenges enables us to shift our perspective and view these experiences as opportunities for personal growth and resilience.

Focusing on those things we are grateful for enables us to let go of negative emotions that can hinder our personal growth and well-being. Gratitude can foster compassion and understanding of others, leading to a greater willingness to empathize with their perspective and understand the context of their actions.

I will admit that it is really challenging to be grateful in moments of pain, loss, and disappointment, but like everything else, gratitude is a skill that can be cultivated and strengthened with practice, gradually becoming more accessible over time.

This Art Therapy intervention uses the "Gratitude tree" print-out provided in this book. You can also draw your own tree, but it must have many branches, lots of roots, and a sun or moon in the background.

Here are the steps for your Art Therapy exercise:

1. In the trunk of the tree, write "I am grateful for..." Use a pen or marker.

2. Write all the things you are grateful for in the branches.

   a. Include pain, loss, and/or disappointments.

   b. Include big and small gratitudes (family and friends *and* chocolate).

   c. Include the specific challenge you've been address-ing—the very issue that led you to explore the Creative Cognitive Therapy Method. This is the monster that you confronted. Maybe for you it is your fear, anger, addiction, or grief.

3. Fill in the ground area below the tree with things that make you feel grounded and rooted.

4. In the circle/sun write the things that make you feel connected to others and the world around you: religion, spirituality, nature...

5. Color in the drawing any way you want. You can use watercolor paints, crayons, markers, or colored pencils.

Art Therapy exercise: Gratitude tree

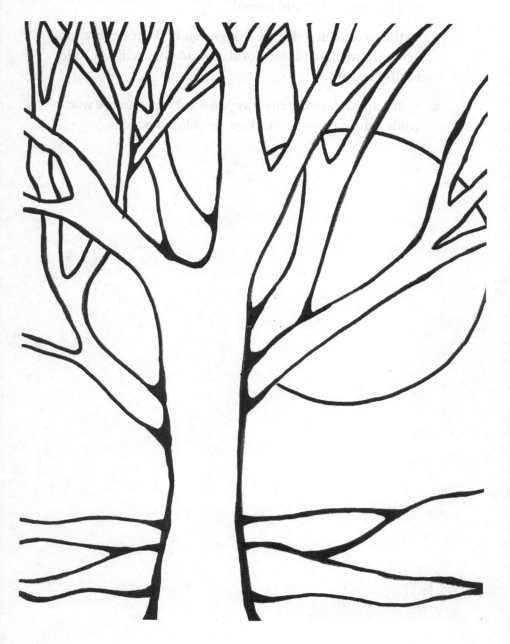

⬇ Art Therapy exercise example: Gratitude tree

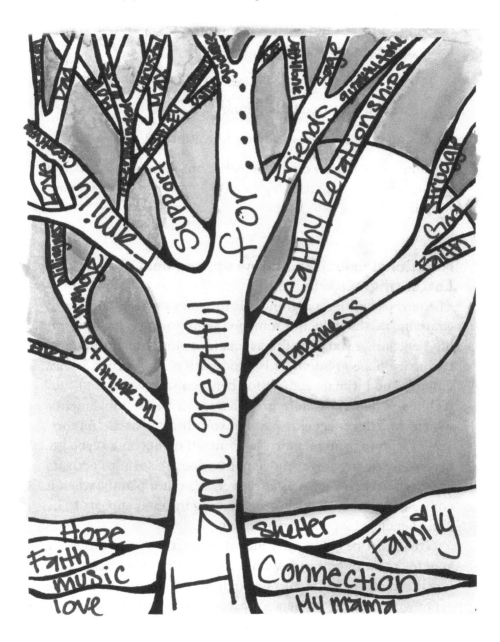

Explanation and discussion prompts

Use the discussion questions to reflect on your experience of drawing your tree and what it communicates, about both your feelings and your journey.

1. How does your mood shift when you focus on gratitude?

2. Are you surprised by anything?

3. Can you continue to add more gratitudes?

Try doing this activity once a month. Continuing the practice of rooting yourself in gratitude can have a powerful effect on your overall well-being.

Additional exercises, follow up, and next steps: Letter of gratitude

The purpose of this assignment is for you to take a moment to contemplate the influence someone significant has had on your life. I encourage you to do this as a handwritten letter, rather than typing it on a computer. This handwritten approach creates a tangible and intimate connection between your words and your feelings. It demands more precise and deliberate movements, which can trigger specific parts of your brain that are important for learning and memory. In contrast, typing on a keyboard, despite involving finger movements, doesn't seem to activate these crucial brain areas as effectively. To put it plainly, when it comes to memory and learning, writing by hand appears to be more beneficial for your brain than typing.[10]

This practice serves as a means to nurture and cultivate a genuine sense of gratitude within you, one that is expressed not just through words but also through the effort you put into the act of writing itself. It offers a space for you to acknowledge and express your gratitude for the invaluable life lessons you may have learned from this person.

Instructions

1. Choose the person. Select someone who holds significance in your life. It could be a family member, friend, mentor, teacher, or even someone who has hurt you but taught you valuable lessons.

2. Reflect on their impact. Take some time to reflect on the positive influence this person has had on your life. Consider the specific ways they have supported, inspired, or taught you important life lessons. Think about how they have shaped your values, beliefs, or personal growth.

3. Start the letter. Begin your letter by expressing your genuine gratitude and explain why they are important to you. Be specific about the actions, qualities, or moments that have made a lasting impression.

4. Acknowledge life lessons. If applicable, acknowledge any challenging experiences or conflicts you have had with this person. Share how these experiences have taught you important lessons and helped you grow as an individual.

5. This step is optional. You can choose to share the letter with the person if you feel it would be appropriate and would be well-received. However, remember that the purpose of this exercise is primarily for your own self-reflection and growth.

My client, Sasha, wrote a letter of gratitude to her cousin, Tina, with whom she'd not spoken in many years. They'd had a falling out just before Sasha's wedding day when Tina pleaded with Sasha not to go through with the marriage. She expressed her worries about Sasha's fiancé's emotional abuse and controlling behavior.

Hey Tina,

It's been way too damn long since we last spoke, and there's something I need to get off my chest. I've been doing some serious thinking about the shit that went down between us, and I gotta say, I'm grateful for what you did.

Remember when you told me I shouldn't marry Marcus? Yeah, back then I thought you were just hating on my happiness, but now I see it differently. You were actually looking out for me. Plus, he turned out to be a real asshole, just like you warned me. I think I even knew that back then, but didn't want to admit it.

I'm reaching out to thank you for always being there, even in the midst of our messed-up dynamics.

With gratitude,
Sasha

Sasha struggled with a clenched jaw and shallow breathing while she read the letter out loud to me. When she finished, she folded up her paper and shoved it into her pocket. Only then did she make eye contact with me. Her eyes were full of tears.

I asked Sasha if she would consider sharing the letter with her cousin. There was a brief pause, as Sasha collected her thoughts before she replied, "Yes, I want to send it to her, but I'm worried that too much time has passed and she won't forgive me."

We then talked about how it's never too late to rebuild a relationship, particularly if a person is willing to acknowledge their own role in the falling out. I assured Sasha that taking responsibility and committing to change could pave the way for healing and reconciliation.

Eckhart Tolle's message encourages us to view the present moment as our friend and ally: "Whatever the present moment contains, accept it as if you had chosen it. Always work with it, not against it. Make it your friend and ally, not your enemy. This will miraculously transform your whole life." We can approach every situation with an open attitude and a willingness to learn and adapt. By doing so, we will cultivate a sense of resilience and strength that will serve us well throughout our lives.

NOTES FOR THERAPISTS

Begin this session by introducing the quotation by Eckhart Tolle and outlining the goals for the session. Take a few moments to revisit the "What you are carrying/holding" drawing assigned as homework. Encourage your client to share what they continue to carry with them and whether their drawing symbolizes the act of letting go or shedding any lingering negative thoughts.

During this sixth session, guide your client through the "Put your crystal ball away" CBT exercise, followed by a discussion. Suggest that your client make some brief notes to refer back to later, or they can choose to write their thoughts in their journal, with the understanding that this option may consume more session time. Additionally, ensure that the "Gratitude tree" exercise is completed within the session.

As homework, assign the "Letter of gratitude." This task offers your client an opportunity to reflect on individuals who have had a positive impact on their life. Acknowledge that some clients may struggle to select just one person, and, in such cases, encourage them to write multiple letters of gratitude if they wish.

It's important to emphasize that personal interpretations and adaptations of the gratitude letter are not only permitted but actively encouraged to cater to the unique needs and experiences of each individual. Stress that the letter need not be exclusively addressed to a living person;

clients can write to someone who has passed away, a beloved pet, a spiritual figure, or even an inanimate object of personal significance. The expression of gratitude knows no bounds in this exercise.

Finally, remind your client that you will review and discuss their gratitude letter during your next meeting.

CHAPTER SEVEN

Seventh Module: Learn to Tolerate Uncomfortable Feelings

Often attributed to the ancient text Tao Te Ching, the Taoist philosopher Lao Tzu is said to have observed: "*New beginnings are often disguised as painful endings.*"[11] This profound statement serves as a poignant reminder that closures and conclusions should not necessarily be viewed through a negative or fearful lens. Instead, they represent an inherent facet of life's ever-turning wheel and can serve as essential catalysts for progress and rejuvenation. By recognizing the potential for the emergence of fresh opportunities within the dissolution of the old, we can approach change with a mindset steeped in positivity and optimism.

This phrase also acknowledges the intrinsic challenges associated with change. It is human nature to find transformation uncomfortable and often to resist it. The sensations of sorrow, frustration, or fear that accompany the relinquishing of the familiar and comfortable are entirely natural. Nevertheless, we are offered the wisdom that these very emotions frequently signal the onset of growth and the seeds of transformation. It is human nature to find transformation uncomfortable and often to resist it. The sensations of sorrow, frustration, or fear that accompany the relinquishing of the familiar and comfortable are entirely natural. Nevertheless, Lao Tzu offers the wisdom that these very emotions frequently signal the onset of growth and the seeds of transformation.

Goals: Learn to tolerate uncomfortable feelings

Today's goal is to develop the valuable skill of tolerating uncomfortable feelings. Life is not always smooth sailing. Sometimes it really sucks! It's natural to want to escape unpleasant and adverse responses to life, leading many people to rely on substances like food, alcohol, drugs, or even excessive social media use in an attempt to numb their emotions. However, these distractions only offer temporary relief.

The more we attempt to avoid or ignore our feelings, the stronger their influence becomes. The quotation "What you resist not only persists, but will grow in size," commonly attributed to Carl Jung, encapsulates this idea, though its definitive source is unclear. Regardless of its origin, the lesson remains: rather than persistently tuning out emotions, it's more beneficial to develop the capacity to tolerate and address them. Essentially, the more we try to evade or dismiss our feelings, the more power they hold over us.

That doesn't mean resigning yourself to a perpetual state of misery. It means recognizing that these emotions are transient and will eventually subside. By leaning into the discomfort, and allowing yourself to experience it without resistance, you gradually become less intimidated by it. Over time, what once seemed overwhelming and terrifying becomes more manageable.

The second goal is to acknowledge and sit with the discomfort of grief or distress or pain. Paradoxically, you're simultaneously building skills to move away from tough feelings. This allows you to avoid getting stuck in them. The ultimate aim is to learn how to control the amount of time you spend grappling with undesirable emotions and discover healthy ways to comfort and soothe yourself without resorting to substances or unhealthy habits.

CBT intervention: Failure is a necessary part of success

Have you ever been so afraid to fail that you remained stuck without even trying? This can apply to many aspects of life.

I had a client who hated their job and dreamed of starting their own business, but the fear of failure kept them stuck in a workplace where they were underpaid and underappreciated. I had another client who desperately wanted to be in a loving relationship, but she was so scared of rejection that she wouldn't put herself out there to date. I even had a client who was so afraid of failure that he refused to play a simple board game with me.

But failure is not the opposite of success—it is a necessary stepping stone. Failure provides valuable lessons and insights that cannot be obtained through success alone. It serves as a teacher, highlighting areas that need improvement, revealing weaknesses, and presenting opportunities for growth. By experiencing failure, you gain firsthand knowledge about what doesn't work. This allows you to adjust your strategies accordingly.

Failure also builds resilience. It tests your resolve and pushes you to persevere despite setbacks. Overcoming failure requires strength and the ability to bounce back from disappointments, which contributes to the development of your tenacity, determination, and ultimately, your character. Moreover, failure often sparks creativity and innovation. When faced with a setback, you are forced to think outside the box, explore alternative solutions, and adapt your approach. This can lead to breakthroughs, unexpected discoveries, and new paths that you may not have considered otherwise.

Think like a scientist. Scientific progress is built upon experimentation, hypothesis testing, and data analysis. In this process, unexpected outcomes are not only anticipated but also embraced. Each failure provides valuable information, helping scientists refine their understanding and refine their methods.

Here is your challenge (to be completed as a writing exercise in your journal):

1. Take one past failure and consider both the misfortune and benefit.

2. What lessons did you learn?

3. How are you a different, stronger, wiser, or more compassionate person now?

Art Therapy exercise: Feeling drawings and guided visualization

For this Art Therapy exercise, three pieces of white paper are needed to create three different drawings. Before beginning with the drawings, I want you to take a moment to think about the uncomfortable emotion that you have been exploring throughout our previous six modules. Whether you are focusing on feelings of anxiety, anger, resentment, restlessness, or depression, I want you to close your eyes and visualize that specific feeling.

What colors do you associate with this emotion? Imagine the shape of this feeling. Does it appear large or small to you? Is it a simple shape or does it consist of intricate and complex lines?

Using the first piece of paper, draw your feeling. Just use colors, lines, and shapes that you visualized. Remember, there is no right or wrong way to express yourself through art. I encourage you to do this fairly quickly, without overthinking it. This should not take more than five minutes to complete.

After completing your first drawing, set it aside, and take a moment to pause. Now, shift your focus to visualizing how you *would like* to feel, which should be in stark contrast to the previous emotion you explored. Close your eyes and allow yourself to envision this new desired feeling. Reflect on what colors resonate with this emotion. Consider whether these shapes are smooth flowing curves or perhaps geometric patterns.

Now, take your second piece of paper and create a drawing that reflects how you want to feel. As with the first drawing, don't overthink this. This should not take you more than five minutes.

For instance, Maurice's first drawing showed his anger with chaotic red, orange, and black lines.

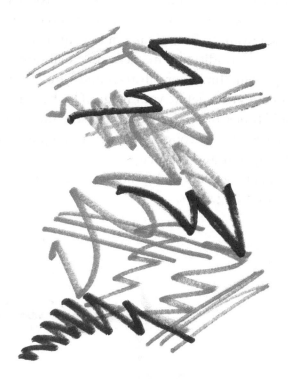

In his second drawing, he switched to expressing gratitude and acceptance using calm green and blue wavy lines.

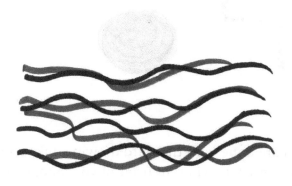

Once you have finished your second drawing, set it aside and take a moment to pause once again. Now, for the third drawing, let's delve into the realm of imagination and envision a magical element that has the power to transform your initial "yucky" feeling into how you want to feel. What would your magic look like? Is it embodied by a traditional magic wand, a vibrant lightning bolt, or perhaps something more abstract and symbolic? Consider the colors and lines that define your magic. Do they radiate with bright and bold tones, or do they consist of soft and subtle hues? Remember that everyone's concept of magic is unique. Using your third piece of paper, draw your magic.

Maurice's magic was simple but bold: he drew a shining star at the top of ascending stairs.

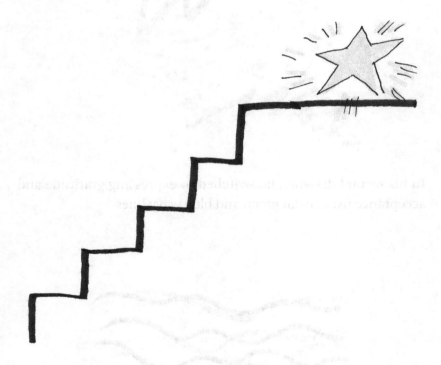

Once you are done with the third drawing, take a moment to arrange all three drawings in front of you. Simply observe the images without passing judgment on whether they are good or bad. Notice any similarities or stark differences between your representation of the "yucky" feeling and your desired state of mind.

Now, let's do a meditative exercise, which includes muscle tension and release. If you're new to meditation, don't worry! Just close your eyes and take a few deep breaths. In through your nose and out through your mouth. Tighten up the muscles throughout your body. Clench your fists, jaw, and buttocks. This might feel strange but hang in there! Envision the shapes and colors from the first drawing gradually expanding to fill your entire body. Hold your breath while you stay here for a few seconds. Allow yourself to fully immerse in the experience. This is supposed to be uncomfortable, but only stay here for five to eight seconds.

Next, take a deep breath in, and as you exhale, imagine your magical element making its appearance. Visualize your magic flowing in and washing away the unpleasant colors and shapes. Allow your magic to erase the yucky feeling (your first drawing) and reveal your desired feeling (your second drawing). As you breathe and your muscles relax, picture your magic as an eraser wiping away the yucky feeling and revealing the desired feeling. Remind yourself that your true feelings are constant but may be obscured by negativity, much like the sun hidden behind storm clouds. Recognize your second drawing as your core self, always present but sometimes waiting to resurface. Take a moment to experience the peace, relaxation, and any other positive feelings that arise from this visualization.

Explanation and discussion prompts

After you finish creating your three drawings, I suggest you arrange them in front of you, forming a series. Take a moment to reflect on your experience throughout the process before diving into the details of each drawing. Remember that, sometimes, the journey is just as important as the finished product.

I also encourage you to examine the differences between your drawings. This practice can help you notice patterns, symbols, or images that may unconsciously surface across your artwork. By the eighth session, these recurring themes often become more noticeable and apparent to you.

Each person's experience of art-making is highly individualized, often reflecting their overall approach to life. For instance, my client Jeremy, who frequently expressed exhaustion and feeling overworked, found the process draining since he was unaccustomed to creating three drawings in one session. In contrast, Cecilia, known for her adventurous nature and openness to new experiences, described the process as exciting, challenging, and ultimately enjoyable. Following the discussion of their experience, I invited them to explore similarities in shapes, colors, or recurring themes that emerged within pairs or even across all three drawings.

If you're interested in exploring your experience more profoundly, you can make use of the following discussion questions to contemplate your three drawings and your experience of the guided visualization. This can aid in gaining a deeper understanding of yourself and how you're constructing your mental wellness toolbox.

1. Describe your experience of making three drawings in a row.

2. Describe the drawings as a series.

3. Do you see any similarities or themes in all the drawings? Or two of the drawings?

4. What are the big differences that you notice between the different drawings?

Also, use the following questions to explore the process of engaging with the guided visualization.

1. What was your experience of muscle tension during the guided visualization?

2. Were you able to visualize your images filling up your body?

3. What physical sensations did you feel when you were visualizing the first drawing (the uncomfortable feeling)?

4. Was there a recognizable shift when you brought in the magic to erase the first image?

5. What physical sensations did you feel when you were visualizing the second drawing (the opposite feeling)?

6. Can you make this visualization a daily routine? If you pair it with something that you already do daily, such as brushing your teeth or getting ready for bed, it will be easier to be consistent.

Engaging in the practice of tensing your muscles and visualizing unpleasant emotions gives you a unique chance to sit with the discomfort that these feelings bring. In your everyday life, you may go to great lengths to avoid feeling such emotions, searching for quick fixes to make them vanish. Nonetheless, it's vital to develop the skill of tolerating these uncomfortable feelings without turning to instant gratification or unhealthy coping methods. Instead of relying on external distractions like drugs, food, angry outbursts, or alcohol as ways to escape or numb these emotions, I encourage my clients to build resilience and emotional tolerance by actively embracing brief moments of discomfort. Through this deliberate practice, a person can gradually expand their capacity to sit with and process these challenging emotions, fostering personal growth and emotional well-being.

I encourage you to practice this visualization every day on your own, and then consider gradually extending the time you spend sitting with those uncomfortable feelings—add a few seconds each day as you hold your breath and tense your muscles. This will help you to further tolerate those moments of feeling uncomfortable. Remember that the more you repeat a behavior like this, the easier it becomes. Behaviors can turn into habits—and habits eventually shape your character.

You might be reluctant to embrace those undesirable emotions because you're scared of getting trapped in fear, sadness, or anger. However, through this art and guided visualization exercise, you've actually created your own "escape button." You've identified a kind of magic that has the potential to transform those unwanted emotions into how you ultimately want to feel. In addition, you've pinpointed what you desire to feel, which is a powerful understanding to help you move forward.

Additional exercises, follow up, and next steps: Praise Poem

Now, let's move on to our second Art Therapy exercise—and yes, you heard that right, there are two distinct exercises in this section. You're under no obligation to undertake them in succession or even on the same day. In fact, taking a few days in between might be quite beneficial, affording you an emotional breather.

But when you feel prepared, we're going to take a slight departure from the drawing and venture into the realm of creative writing. Your task is to use the prompts on the template to compose a poem that reflects on the past while embracing an image of hope for the future. This exercise will allow you to reflect upon memories, challenges, and growth achieved throughout your life. While acknowledging the weight of the past, this poem will also serve as a source of hope. It will encourage you to envision a brighter future, embracing the power of transformation and evolution.

As an example, below is *my* personal "Praise Poem." Even the Art Therapist gets creative and personal from time to time! I wrote this poem during the year I reconnected with my now-husband after 30 years. We were high school friends but lost touch when we went to college. We met again after the ending of my 20-year marriage, and I'd returned to my hometown for my father's heart surgery. It was comforting to date someone who understood my references and shared mutual friends. However, I struggle with recalling many memories because there was a lot of pot smoking during those high school days! While I wish I could remember more, I am grateful for the opportunity to create new memories with him.

> *Praise to the past that returns to teach me.*
> *Praise to the prom date who returns to my life*
> *as an old comfort but with new wisdom.*
> *Praise to the new home where I live on my*
> *own and have created by myself.*
> *Praise to the smell of cut grass on summer mornings.*
> *Praise to the ocean lined with Italian cypress*
> *trees that look like a Van Gogh painting.*
> *Praise to my grandmother's cooking that takes me*
> *back to a place that I can no longer return.*
> *Praise to the color red that I can now see so*
> *clearly without altered perception.*
> *Praise to the clouded memories that I can barely see,*
> *like Everest shrouded white and snow and mist.*
> *Although darkness may gather, love will be*
> *there now and in my lost memories.*

It is powerful to acknowledge, process, and navigate challenging emotions without succumbing to them. Instead of avoiding or denying hard feelings, you can embrace the power to transform what's been difficult to face, fostering resilience and cultivating a more desirable emotional state. "New beginnings are often disguised as painful endings": facing hard emotions can create a new emotional landscape.

⊕ PRAISE POEM

Praise to the past that returns to teach me.

Praise to the. . . . .

. . . .
Person

who . . . .

. . . .
Describe why/how they are important

Praise to the. . . . .

. . . .
Place

where . . . .

. . . .
Describe

Praise to the smell of . . . .

. . . .
Smell

that. . . . .

. . . .
Describe

Praise to . . . .

. . . .
Something about myself that I do not particularly like

⬇ Praise to the. . . . .

. . . .
Body of water

where . . . .

. . . .
Describe

Praise to the . . . .

. . . .
Food

that. . . . .

. . . .
Describe

Praise to the color. . . . .

. . . .
Color

that. . . . .

. . . .
Describe

Although darkness may gather . . . .

. . . .
Something hopeful about the future

NOTES FOR THERAPISTS

At the outset of this session, have your client read their gratitude letter aloud and encourage them to express any thoughts or emotions that surfaced during the writing or while reading it to you. Additionally, engage in a conversation with them about the potential advantages of delivering the letter to its intended recipient. It's essential to recognize that some individuals may find it challenging to deliver this letter because of the recipient's absence, whether due to passing away or no longer being part of their life. In some cases, the letter may have been written to an animal, a spiritual entity, or an inanimate object.

In the seventh session, guide your client through the "Failure is a necessary part of success" (reframing failure) CBT exercise, followed by a discussion. Also, ensure that all three drawings of the Art Therapy exercise are completed, and guide them through the visualization exercise during the session.

For homework, strongly recommend that your client practice the guided visualization exercise. Encourage them to gradually increase the duration of breath-holding and muscle tension each time, stressing that breath-holding should not exceed 10 seconds at most. It can be more effective if they designate a specific time each day for this visualization. Allow them to choose the timing that feels most comfortable as it can aid in establishing a daily routine that, when consistently maintained for a few weeks, can eventually evolve into a healthy habit.

You will also assign the "Praise Poem" as additional homework and offer your client the sentence completion worksheet to guide their writing. Emphasize that they should bring their completed poem to the next session for further discussion.

I recommend that you, as the therapist, consider composing your own Praise Poem. Sharing your own poem can foster a sense of connection with your client, but it's important to strike a balance by ensuring it is honest without delving into overly personal details. There's a fine line between sharing common ground and overwhelming them with personal information. Providing an example can clarify the poem's structure, expectations, and its purpose.

CHAPTER EIGHT

Eighth Module:
Gain Acceptance

Once I saw the words written *"I never knew how strong I was until I had to forgive someone who wasn't sorry, and accept an apology I never received."* I have no idea who said it, but it really stuck with me. I understand this quotation to be saying that forgiving someone who isn't sorry can be particularly challenging because it may feel like you're letting them off the hook or excusing their behavior. This really resonated with me. I believe that forgiveness is not about absolving the other person of their actions or condoning what they did. It's about releasing yourself from the pain that's holding you back and keeping you from moving toward growth. On the healing journey, it's important to embrace the inevitability of fear and pain as integral aspects of life. Whether it is emotional or physical, we instinctively avoid pain at all costs—and waiting for someone else to apologize or make things right takes us out of the driver's seat of our own well-being. Achieving acceptance of *what is* requires effort and conscious steps.

Goals: Accepting that pain is a part of life
One crucial step for healing is to recognize that multiple realities and perspectives exist for every situation. We must intentionally seek a shift from what we once thought was true. This shift in perspective can assist us in realizing that the pain may not have

been inflicted intentionally, but rather it may have been an un-intended consequence of someone else's actions.

Another essential aspect of this acceptance involves forgive-ness. Embracing forgiveness doesn't mean denying the hurt we've experienced or excusing bad behavior. Instead, it releases us from carrying destructive anger. Sometimes we just have to let some of that shit go. Unfortunately, many individuals cling to their pain for prolonged periods, allowing it to shape their identity and influ-ence their interactions with others. You have likely encountered individuals who exude constant anger. However, by embracing forgiveness, we reclaim the power to determine which emotions define us.

The final goal today is to be advocates for ourselves by putting into practice the art of seeking help. This can prove challenging as we often fear being perceived as weak or burdensome. How-ever, I encourage you to reframe your perspective on this matter. Consider that we all inherently desire to be helpful and experience the positive emotions that come with it. When you ask others for support, view it as granting them an opportunity to be benevolent rather than burdening them. In fact, by not seeking help, you might inadvertently deny others the chance to feel genuinely good about themselves through acts of kindness and assistance. Embracing this mindset can foster a supportive and interconnected community where everyone benefits from giving and receiving help.

CBT intervention: Forgiveness

Forgiveness is a powerful act that should not be mistaken for con-doning bad behavior; rather, it shields us from the corrosive grip of anger that can consume and harm us. Oftentimes, those who hurt us did not intend to inflict pain, yet we may find ourselves wounded in the aftermath of their thoughtless or self-centered words and actions. Choosing to forgive demonstrates a remark-able strength of character, a deep sense of love for ourselves and others, and a recognition of the interconnections that bind us all.

By letting go of resentment and embracing forgiveness, we create space for healing, compassion, and growth.

I would like to share a personal story of pain, loss, and forgiveness that profoundly impacted my life. My marriage lasted for two decades, and during the initial twelve years, my husband was a kind and devoted father. He consciously avoided alcohol, not wanting to follow the path of his many family members who struggled with alcoholism. However, when he turned 40, he made the decision to start drinking, which unfortunately led to the deterioration of our relationship. His judgment became clouded by alcohol, and he made a series of regrettable decisions, including spending our life savings on a movie he was making. That was the final straw and the end of our marriage.

Naturally, I felt anger and resentment. I saw myself as a victim, believing he had betrayed our family. I blamed myself for trusting him with our finances.

Over time, the burden of that anger became too heavy for me to bear. I needed to get out of my own head. Desperately searching for a different perspective, I tried to comprehend things from his perspective. I came to the realization that he never intended to harm us. In his mind, the movie was a stepping stone to financial success. He genuinely believed it would be a blockbuster hit. Despite his poor choices fueled by alcohol, he never meant to inflict pain on our children or me.

With this newfound perspective, I began to let go of much of my anger, though, to be honest, a trace of resentment still remains, and I continue to work on its dissolution. Embracing forgiveness is not about pretending the past never happened; it's acknowledging the pain, learning from it, and moving forward. Sometimes very slowly.

Without forgiveness those feelings would have warped my view of the world, making it hard for me to trust anyone again. I'd be scared of opening up to others, and that's just not the life I wanted. Realizing that my ex's actions were not driven by malicious intent allowed me to view that particular event as an isolated incident rather than a representation of the entire human experience. People are complex, and we all make mistakes. Finding forgiveness was a gift to myself, not for him. No longer restrained by the past, I found the courage to open my heart to build strong healthier relationships with friends, family, and eventually a new partner.

Forgiving others releases us from the burden of anger and resentment. Holding onto negative emotions is exhausting, both mentally and physically, and it hinders personal growth and relationships. Forgiveness is like taking back the keys to your happiness and saying, "Sorry, you can't drive me crazy anymore!"

Below are some questions to help you explore why forgiveness is important:

1. Is there someone who has hurt you—someone whom you haven't been able to forgive? Put yourself in their shoes.

    a. Did they intend to hurt you? Or were you hurt in the wake of their bad decisions and selfishness?

    b. What could they have been thinking/intending by the behavior that hurt you?

2. Who is being punished by holding onto the anger/ resentment?

    a. If you continue to hold onto this hurt, how might it warp your view of the world and other people?

3. What would you lose if you forgave them? What would you gain?

4. What would it take to find forgiveness and let go?

Art Therapy exercise: Create, destroy, rebuild

This Art Therapy exercise will take you through multiple steps as you experience your art transforming from something difficult to something more hopeful. You will have the opportunity to express your uncomfortable feelings through the language of color, shapes, and lines. You will talk to those feelings, dismantle them, then rebuild to find something new and encouraging in your new foundation.

Let's walk through the steps together.

Draw your uncomfortable feeling with crayons. This is the same struggle you have been focused on since Chapter One. Take a moment and think about what your feeling might look like. Is it ugly? Then find some ugly colors. Is it sharp and menacing? Then try drawing the emotion as sharp, jagged lines, and unsettling colors. Perhaps it's a tangled, chaotic mess inside you? In that case, you may want to create scribbly, overlapping lines and shapes. Remember, there's no right or wrong way to visually express your inner turmoil. Don't overthink it; just let it out. Unleash that putrid feeling onto the paper, as if you're vomiting it out!

Example: Uncomfortable feeling—"Out of control"

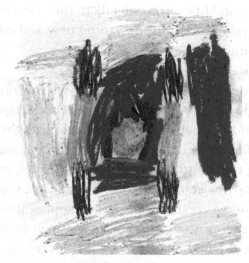

Example: Uncomfortable feeling—"Sad"

While some clients develop a strong attachment to their uncomfortable feelings (and the drawings of those feelings), many find these depictions unpleasant and unsatisfying. If you find yourself among the latter group, you probably won't offer much resistance as I suggest crumpling up your creation. Yes, you heard me right—crumple it up! Just like our feelings, nothing is permanent, and this act serves as a poignant reminder of that truth. As you are crumpling, really be present with the experience. Listen to the sounds. Feel the sharp edges of the paper. Notice if the image has smeared or changed in any way.

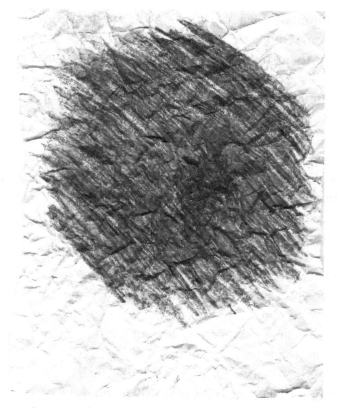

Example: Crumpled uncomfortable feeling—"Out of control"

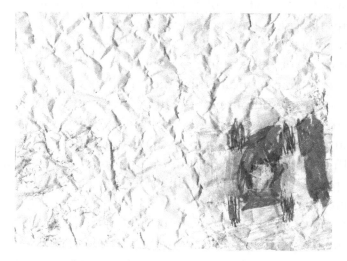

Example: Crumpled uncomfortable feeling—"Sad"

If you found the idea of crumpling up your drawing a bit peculiar, brace yourself, because I might sound really crazy now! Take a moment to open up your crumpled drawing and gaze at it. Now, here's the kicker—speak to it. Yup, you heard that right! You can say it out loud if you're alone, or simply do it silently if others are around.

Feel free to vent your frustrations or your confusion. You may want to curse at it, "You've messed up my life!" Alternatively, maybe you're grappling with questions, and you can ask, "Why are you always here?" Seriously, anything goes. This exercise is your personal outlet, an opportunity to let it all out and confront those feelings head-on. So go ahead, speak your mind, and breathe into the release it brings. There's no judgment here—only a safe space to confront what's been troubling you.

Once you've expressed yourself to the drawing, it's time for another round of crumpling. Pay attention to the sounds and texture of the paper as you crumple it for the second time. Typically, the sound is a bit quieter, and you'll notice the paper becoming softer to the touch as its fibers are pulled apart.

Without delay, open it up, gently placing it flat on the table, and examine it closely. Has it undergone any changes? Is the paper now smaller than when you started? Does it carry a new texture? Perhaps the colors have mixed or even flaked off?

Say something to you drawing for the second time. You can repeat what you said earlier, or maybe there's something different you wish to communicate this time.

Repeat the crumpling of the drawing for a third time. Continue to notice the sounds, textures, and changes. It might come as a surprise, but what you're actually doing here is practicing mindfulness. Yes, that's right, mindfulness can be as simple as this—paying close attention to all those little details and engaging all your different senses.

Let's have one final interaction with the crappy feeling. Now that you have damaged your drawing, it's time to take it one step further and destroy it completely. Tear it into many little pieces.

Then, divide the ripped-up pieces into two equal piles. Keep one pile and discard the other half. Here is where the Art Therapy exercise becomes a metaphor for life.

You may be tempted to toss it all in the garbage, but I'm urging you to retain some of those ugly feelings. This is art as metaphor. Rather than trying to erase or ignore those feelings, we're going to explore ways to integrate them into your lived experience. These emotions can be transformed from a perceived personal failing into a source of strength. For now, go ahead and discard one half, while holding onto the rest, but set it aside momentarily; we'll return to it shortly.

Changing our focus, shift gears and concentrate on the positive. Think of a word that is diametrically opposed to the crummy feeling you just drew and ripped up. For instance, if the feeling you drew was "anxiety," maybe your opposite word would be "calm" or "control" or "content." It will be different for everyone. Choose the word that works for you.

Now, it's time to select a colored piece of paper that resonates with the positive word you've chosen. Maybe that is the opposite color of the ugly colors you used to draw your yucky feelings.

Once you've selected the correct colored paper, write your word on it. But don't stop at just writing it once—write it repeatedly, letting it fill the space in different ways. Write it big. Write is small. Print it. Write it in script or big block letters. Experiment by turning the paper around, letting your word sprawl in various directions. You can even flip the paper over and write on the back side. This repetition isn't just random; it's what makes the word truly powerful.

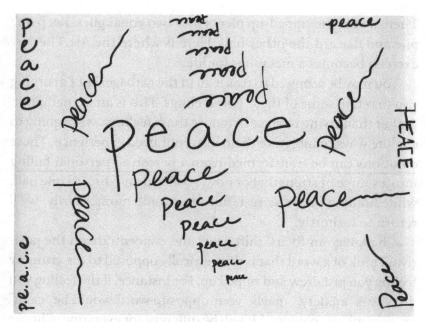

Example: Empowering word on colored paper.
Opposite of "Out of control" is "Peace"

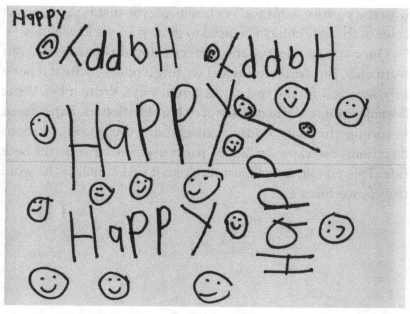

Example: Empowering word on colored paper.
Opposite of "Sad" is "Happy"

When you have no more room to write, fold your paper in half. Really crease that fold, because you are going to intentionally rip the paper into two pieces.

Recall the moment when you haphazardly tore up that dreadful feeling drawing? Now, we're taking a different approach—this time, it's all about focus, precision, and purpose. With the first drawing, you tossed out half of those unpleasant emotions. However, the goal now isn't to discard a comforting feeling; it's about sharing it with others!

Picture this: eventually, you'll be handing over half of that paper to someone else as an offering. Imagine saying to them, "Can I offer you some (insert the positive word you chose)?" Whether that someone is in the room with you at this very moment or if you decide to share it tomorrow, the act of giving "acceptance," "comfort," or "love" is undeniably gratifying. Trust me, it may sound a tad whimsical, but it's a genuinely lovely gesture—one that not only makes you feel good but also resonates with those on the receiving end.

Finally, you are going to gather up those ripped up pieces of yucky feeling and the half piece of colored paper and collage them back together in any manner you want. You can fold or rip the colored paper more, or you can leave it as one piece. But the exercise is to combine both the yucky and the positive together. Find a way to integrate them. You can use the colored paper to hide or protect the negative feeling or you can use both to make an entirely new piece of art. The metaphor here is that our lives will have both positive and tough feelings, and it is our job to find ways to embrace all of it.

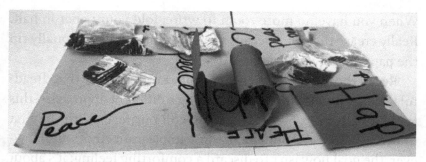

Example: Collage of uncomfortable and empowering
feelings—"Out of control" and "Peace"

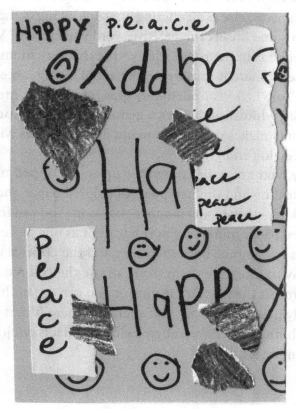

Example: Collage of uncomfortable and
empowering feelings—"Sad" and "Happy"

Here is a summary of all the steps to complete this Art Therapy exercise:

1. Use crayons to draw your uncomfortable feeling.

2. Crumple up your drawing.

3. Uncrumple the drawing and talk to it (do that three times).

4. Rip it up.

5. Keep half and throw away half.

6. Write your opposite, empowering feeling on a piece of colored paper.

7. Fold, crease, and tear the colored paper in half.

8. Create a collage using the yucky, uncomfortable ripped up feeling drawing and the empowering feeling on colored paper.

Explanation and discussion prompts

Phew, that journey encompassed quite a number of steps, and it's likely that it felt rather intense. Take a breather and, when you feel ready, spend some time thinking about the questions that come next. They are like little keys that can unlock a deeper level of insight as you put pen to paper in your reflective journal. If you're on this journey with a therapist or coach, these questions can be the starting point for some truly eye-opening conversations. Don't hesitate to explore them in any order that feels right for you—you don't have to tackle them all if you don't want to. Their purpose is to spark meaningful conversations with yourself and gently guide you into some soul-searching that really matters.

Pause and reflect on what you said to your drawing each time you crumpled it. Did you find yourself repeating the same statement, or did it evolve over time? Just like your drawing went through transformations with each crumple, your words may have also undergone shifts in response to your feelings. This exercise is not only about the physical changes in the drawing but also about the emotional journey you embarked on while engaging with it.

1. Describe your process.

2. What did your drawing look like and how did it change when you crumpled it?

3. What did you say to it? Did that change or stay the same each time?

4. How did it feel to let some go? Keep some?

5. Describe the final piece and how it is different from the original.

6. Did you feel a physical change?

Additional exercises, follow up, and next steps: What you are carrying/holding (3rd time)

Cast your mind back to the distant memory of the second module, where I prompted you to illustrate what you were clutching onto. In that moment, you chose an object to symbolize your ANTs (Automatic Negative Thoughts). Perhaps it was a cube, a brick, or even a ball, an emblem of the weight you bore. You depicted yourself carrying these as mental burdens. Then, fast-forward to the fifth module, where you portrayed yourself releasing and liberating some of those ANTs that had been your constant companions.

Now, let's circle back to that same Art Therapy exercise once more, this time with a subtle twist. Without sneaking a peek at your original drawings, sketch yourself shouldering those burdens now. This time, start by drawing a line to signify the ground, and imagine yourself standing on it. Similar to the initial two drawings, you'll illustrate the ANTs you continue to hold and the ones you're willing and capable of relinquishing.

Pause for a moment. Consider whether any fresh ANTs have

surfaced that warrant inclusion in your drawing. Also, check in with yourself to see whether there might be old ANTs that you're prepared to bid farewell to at this juncture.

This exercise revisits familiar territory but we are going to add a new dimension. You are going to add some flowers, plants, bushes, or trees to your drawing. The plants are a metaphor for the intentions you're looking to nurture and cultivate in your life. In other words, these are your PANTs (Present Affirming Nurturing Thoughts).

In this process, you're embracing the concept of growth and transformation. Much like how a seed germinates and blossoms into a full-grown plant, your intentions have the potential to flourish and become a significant part of your reality. By choosing to depict these intentions through drawings, you're acknowledging their importance and setting the stage for their development. Here are just a few examples of intentions that you may want to plant and cultivate:

Self-Care	Creativity	Adventure
Gratitude	Connection	Patience
Confidence	Courage	Simplicity
Kindness	Resilience	Empowerment
Mindfulness	Health	

ERIN'S STORY

Against the backdrop of green grass, Erin positioned herself surrounded by five vibrant red flowers and two trees featuring green and brown hues. This marked a notable shift as Erin introduced color into her drawings for the first time. In her description, Erin revealed that the elements she incorporated symbolized her intentions: staying connected to her culture and family, prioritizing time in nature, and cultivating a daily practice of gratitude.

In her third iteration of the exercise, Erin depicting herself holding onto an increased number of items, notably a circle grasped in her hand labeled "JOB." Just that week Erin had been offered, and accepted, a job!

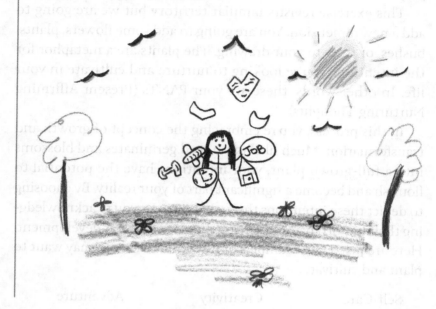

While the quotation "I never knew how strong I was until I had to forgive someone who wasn't sorry, and accept an apology I never received" may seem to address forgiving others and accepting unoffered apologies, it carries a deeper resonance that can be translated into the journey of self-forgiveness. It speaks to the strength required for both acts and underscores the powerful connection between forgiving others and embracing self-forgiveness.

The realization of strength mentioned in the quotation can extend to the realization of inner strength and resilience in the context of self-forgiveness. Just as it takes strength to forgive someone who doesn't express remorse, it also takes courage to face our own mistakes, make amends, and move forward with self-compassion.

The quotation guides us to let go, which is essential in both forgiving others and forgiving oneself. By forgiving someone and accepting an apology never received, we learn to release the emotional burden tied to the situation. Similarly, self-forgiveness often involves letting go of self-blame and allowing ourselves to heal.

NOTES FOR THERAPISTS

Begin this session by sharing the forgiveness quotation and clarifying the session's objectives. Have your client read their Praise Poem aloud and engage them in a discussion about their experience and insights.

During your session, guide your client through the CBT exercise "Forgiveness," focused on understanding other people's intentions and finding forgiveness. Ensure that you complete all eight steps of the Art Therapy exercise together and follow it up with a discussion to thoroughly review their experience with the exercise.

For homework, assign your client the task of drawing "What you are carrying/holding" for the third time. Emphasize the importance of adding any intentions they are planting, along with noting any new Automatic Negative Thoughts (ANTs) they are letting go of. Remind your client to bring this drawing to your ninth session so that you can delve into a discussion about their personal growth and progress.

CHAPTER NINE

Ninth Module:
Starting to See Real Change

In our busy lives, it's crucial to sometimes stop and think about where we are and how far we've come, especially when we're feeling stuck or unsure about our future. Think of it like taking a pit stop on your journey. Danielle LaPorte, who writes about personal growth and spirituality, once said, *"Pull over to the side of your journey and look at how far you've come."*[12] She reminds us to appreciate our accomplishments. This message requires knowing yourself, being creative, and recognizing your growth. It is essential to acknowledge the things you're good at and passionate about. Recognizing how far you've come can boost your confidence and motivation. It gives you the courage to keep going on your journey. And by doing this, you'll gain a better perspective, feel more grateful, and find the strength to move forward.

Goals: Seeing real change
Nurturing our new intentions, behaviors, and perspectives

Changing our perspective, intentions, and behaviors has the potential to initiate significant transformation in our lives. By shifting our perspective, we alter the way we perceive challenges and setbacks, enabling us to view them as opportunities for growth and learning. Concurrently, setting clear and positive intentions directs our focus toward our desired goals. Rather than simply reacting to external events, setting intentions serves as a guide that molds our actions and choices, aligning them with our aspirations and desired outcomes.

It is important to understand the difference between reaction and response. In the context of interpersonal conflicts, reactions are often fueled by emotions and can exacerbate situations. A reaction typically stems from the need to shield our ego, propelling us into defensive and attacking mode. Often, when someone says something that hurts us, we want to hurt them back. The impulse to retaliate might be strong, yet this approach seldom resolves conflicts; rather, it escalates issues and damages relationships.

In contrast, opting for a well-considered response demands effort. Responding entails a deliberate pause, a breath to ground oneself, and a critical question: "What words or actions can I employ, stemming from a place of compassion, to positively reinforce this relationship?"

Choosing to respond, and not react, is not easy, because more often than not, we just want to fight for our position of "being right." Yet, within this challenge lies the potential for growth because by choosing to respond and not react, we are setting healthy intentions—intentions that dictate our behaviors. Repeated behaviors gradually evolve into patterns. Over time, these patterns solidify into habits, ultimately shaping our character. The pivotal question arises: what facets of character do you aspire to embody? And it all stems from choice—your choice to respond with compassion.

CBT intervention: Put on your seatbelt before the car accident

It would not make sense for you to try and put your seatbelt on in the middle of a car accident—that would be nearly impossible. What makes much more sense is that you put on your seatbelt every time you get into the car in case an accident happens. That way you have prepared yourself.[13]

Daily healthy habits are essential, not just during tough times. What you regularly do becomes your go-to during challenging times. Just like a daily glass of wine might turn into a crutch under stress, consistently jogging will make you more likely want to go out for a run when faced with difficulties.

> My client, Lane, is a 27-year-old, non-binary tech engineer. They have a high-paying, high-stress job. In the past four months they have been having seemingly random panic attacks. Sometimes the panic comes in the middle of the workday, other times it wakes them up from a deep sleep at night. Lane mentioned trying a breathing technique they discovered on TikTok, attempting it each time anxiety ramped up. However, despite their efforts, the technique hasn't proven effective.

The challenge with practicing self-care or using distraction techniques solely during moments of anxiety is that the new behavior can become closely associated with the undesired feeling, in this case, anxiety or panic. This connection forms because when we consistently pair two behaviors, they tend to fuse in our minds over time.

Consider this scenario: If I habitually grab a coffee and a scone each time I start my commute to work, I'll eventually link driving with eating. As a result, it becomes difficult to drive without craving a treat.

> In Lane's case, an unexpected connection has formed between panic and deep breathing techniques. Rather than quelling panic, focusing on their breath now unintentionally amplifies their panic. This occurs because Lane's brain associates deep breathing with panic due to consistent pairing. The result is counterproductive to Lane's desired outcome.
>
> A more effective approach involves Lane regularly practicing deep breathing techniques in a calm, secure environment. This consistent practice educates their brain and body on relaxation

and helps them to maintain a lower baseline of anxiety. Consequently, when anxiety and panic now escalate, Lane can employ deep breathing techniques, and their brain recognizes it as a signal of safety and relaxation.

What are you willing to do today to create healthy routines for when times get tough?

Art Therapy exercise: What my hands hold

This Art Therapy exercise offers a profound opportunity to reflect on your initial starting point in this journey, chart your current trajectory, and contemplate the character traits that you want to define your identity.

The first step is to draw an outline of both your left and right hands, using a black pen or marker. If outlining using your non-dominant hand proves challenging, consider asking someone to help you outline your dominant hand.

Your left hand symbolizes the things you've clung to in the past, while your right hand embodies the things you choose to hold onto in the present and future. You might be wondering, "Why is the left hand the past and the right hand the future?" My rationale is that in English-speaking and reading societies, we naturally read from left to right. Consequently, when we examine a drawing or painting, elements on the left tend to precede those on the right. Essentially, the images on the left often evoke a sense of the past or present, while those on the right project a feeling of the future. Naturally, this perspective would vary in cultures that follow reading patterns from right to left or from top to bottom.

Now, keeping this in mind, let's start with your left hand. Take a moment to reflect on all those limiting beliefs and behaviors that you've held onto, the ones that have kept you feeling fearful and stuck. Think about the thoughts, behaviors, and traits that represent these limitations, and use words, symbols, and images to draw them in the outline of your left hand.

Alright, time to give your right hand some attention. This time, envision the thoughts, behaviors, and character traits that you aspire to possess to become the version of yourself that you feel would make your life more joy-filled. These are the qualities that will propel you forward. Consider which words, colors, and images will symbolize and depict these positive attributes, and draw them within the outline of your right hand. This exercise will help you visualize the path toward self-improvement and personal growth.

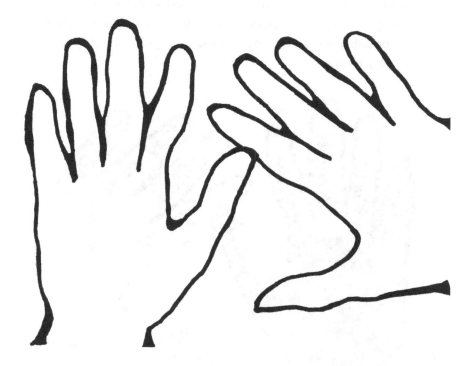

I used to conduct this exercise regularly while leading groups at drug treatment centers, and it consistently brought positive results for my clients. One memorable example involved Becky, who was three months sober from heroin addiction. She was grappling with a profound sense of shame, both in terms of how she had treated others and how she felt about herself.

On her left hand, she inscribed "anger," "betrayal," "regret," "selfishness," and "dishonesty" from pinky to thumb. To accentuate these negative traits, she adorned her left palm with a rain cloud and painted her entire hand red.

In striking contrast, her right hand became a canvas for transformation. Starting with her thumb and moving to her pinky, she wrote "love," "honesty," "pride," "selflessness," and "self-respect." On her right palm, she drew a cloud and a rainbow. This vivid representation captured the profound shift toward positive attributes and self-improvement, while leaving room on the unpainted parts of her hand as a space for new possibilities, all of which marked a significant step in her recovery journey.

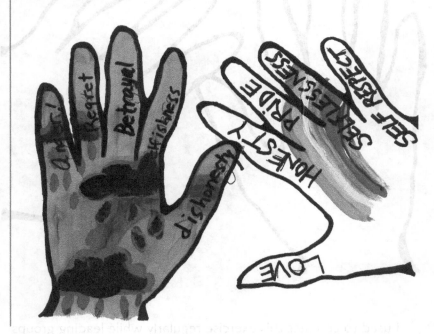

Explanation and discussion prompts

By contrasting the left and right hands, this Art Therapy technique vividly illustrates the difference between our negative and positive attributes, acting as a potent reminder that change and improvement are within reach.

This technique enabled Becky to confront her shame head-on, take responsibility for her choices, and move toward self-improvement. By visually transforming the negative traits drawn onto her left hand into positive ones on her right, she embarked on a path of healing and self-forgiveness.

To delve deeper, consider employing the following questions as a guide. You're welcome to jot down your responses in a journal for a reflective solo journey. On the other hand (pun intended!), you might find it helpful to share your artwork with someone else and talk about it with them. After all, sometimes a heartfelt conversation can uncover hidden truths and perspectives.

1. What came up for you while you were creating this art?

2. Are you surprised by anything that you were holding onto in the past or present?

3. How does it feel to look at this drawing now?

4. How would this drawing have been different if you had done it before you started using this method?

5. Based on this drawing, what behaviors or thoughts might you need to change?

6. What are you most looking forward to in regard to your future?

Writing/journal exercise: Best Possible Self

The "Best Possible Self" (BPS) exercise can be used to increase optimism. This writing exercise requires you to envision yourself in an imaginary future in which everything has turned out in the most optimal way. Picture your life the way you always imagined it would be. You have achieved the things you wanted. You are highly respected, admired, and loved. You are living your dream life. In this scenario, you are the star of your own show—this is your Best Possible Self.

Before I walk you through the process, I want to share the exciting part: research has shown envisioning your Best Possible Self can significantly enhance your mood and overall well-being.[14] Studies have revealed that imagining your BPS can also make you more optimistic about your life journey.[15] And what's even more intriguing is that this boost in optimism happens independently from the mood improvement that the exercise brings. In other words, it's a two-for-one deal: better mood right now and a sunnier outlook for later in life.

To begin, find a quiet place with no distractions, and give yourself at least 30 minutes where you will not be interrupted. As you embark on this expressive journey, grammar and punctuation are not your concern; the spotlight is on pouring out your thoughts and emotions. Dive into each of the seven prompts, dedicating a minimum of five minutes to each. The paper, not the digital screen, is your canvas, as there's a unique connection between handwriting and your brain's creative flow. You may want to have several sheets of paper available for this exercise, because you will be writing at least seven sentences.

Picture yourself having achieved the things you want in life. (It's important to note these should not be total fantasy—for example, do not imagine yourself winning a Nobel Prize for literature unless you have written an exceptionally well-received novel! Imagine that you've harnessed your full potential, reaching the peak of your abilities, and making your desired accomplishments a reality. You are your ultimate self; you are living the dream— YOUR DREAM!

Start with...

1. Write about your perfect home: Where is it located, and what's the neighborhood like? Is it in the city or the countryside, by the ocean, mountains, suburbs, or desert? Are you in a house, apartment, condo, or something more

unique like a boat? Share a bit about your furniture and the things you've filled your space with. How does this setting make you feel?

2. What's keeping you busy? Delve into the world of your career and leisure pursuits. Detail your activities, tasks, and objectives. Are you often indoors or outside? Explore how these activities contribute to your well-being and overall happiness. Moreover, consider the broader impact: How do your activities contribute toward making the world a better place?

3. Who are the key players in your life—family, friends, coworkers, pets, and even the occasional stranger? How do these individuals inspire you, show respect, care for you, or express their love? In return, how do you inspire, respect, care for, and love them? Who forms your tribe, your trusted team, and your unwavering support system?

4. What's on your plate? Not just in terms of food and drinks, but also the other things you're consuming—medications, substances, news, and entertainment. Dive into your culinary preferences, detailing the types of foods and beverages you savor and their origins. Describe how everything that you are nourishing yourself with is a conscious choice toward a healthier and happier you.

5. What are you listening to? Is it music, sounds of nature, conversations, podcasts, the excitement of games, or the chatter of the TV? What fills your ears and surrounds you in a symphony of sounds? Do you hear a train in the distance, evening crickets through an open window, or a steady beat pulsing from your headphones? How do those sounds inspire or relax you?

6. What are you doing to be in service of others? How do you take your talents and passions and make the world a better

place? How do you show love and support to your friends, family, and strangers?

7. What is your emotional state? Describe the different feelings you have and where they come from.

After completing the exercise, reflect and then answer the following questions:

1. What came up for you while you were creating this art?

2. Are you surprised by anything that you are holding onto in the past or present?

3. How does it feel to look at this drawing now?

4. How would this drawing have been different if you had done it before we started working together?

5. Did it motivate or inspire you?

6. Does it make you want to make changes?

7. On a scale from 0 (not at all) to 10 (absolutely!), how achievable does this life seem?

8. How can you start living this life now?

9. What small steps can you make today toward your Best Possible Self?

This module demonstrates that recognizing how far you've come is crucial for continuing your wellness journey. And you've indeed covered a substantial distance on this path. Do you sense the transformations within yourself? Can you see how far you've come? The journey toward self-improvement is an ongoing one, and it's not always a walk in the park. Honestly, it is easier to remain complacent and stuck in our own fears. However, easy only feels good on the surface—it rarely feels good deep down. I am proud of you for all the work you have done. "Pull over to the side of your journey and look at how far you've come": appreciate your accomplishments.

And let's keep this momentum going...

NOTES FOR THERAPISTS

As always, start this session with the quotation and the goals. Then move on to reviewing the homework from session eight. Encourage your clients to share which plants they drew and how those are related to the intentions they are cultivating. Also, ask if they feel that their burden is getting lighter, remaining the same, or getting heavier. Ask if they are starting to see any positive changes in their life, their mood, and/or their relationships. In fact, encourage your client to ask the significant people in their life if they have noticed any positive change in their behavior or mood.

During this session, ensure that your client completes the CBT exercise about implementing healthy habits on a daily basis. In addition, complete the "What my hands hold" Art Therapy exercise.

Assign the "Best Possible Self" writing exercise as homework. It's crucial to emphasize the importance of taking their time with this task and incorporating lots of specifics and details. This exercise can be a powerful tool in promoting positive thinking and envisioning a better future.

CHAPTER TEN

Tenth Module:
Declare Your Independence

Author Brené Brown has been open about her struggles with anxiety and depression. She says: *"When you get to a place where you understand that love and belonging (your worthiness) is a birthright and not something you have to earn,* anything *is possible!"*[16] In her book *The Gifts of Imperfection,*[17] she speaks about the importance of being honest when we refer to our mental health issues. She emphasizes the need for self-care and setting boundaries to protect our emotional well-being. Brown's quotation points to the importance of understanding that our value as human beings is inherent and not something that we have to earn. Many people struggle with feelings of worthlessness, believing that they have to prove themselves or earn the love and acceptance of others. This mindset can be damaging and limit our potential in life. However, when we recognize that our worthiness is not dependent on external factors, such as our achievements or others' opinions of us, we free ourselves to pursue our dreams and live our lives to the fullest.

Goals: Declaring yourself now independent from your fear

- Living your best possible life.

- Becoming the person you were meant to be.

- Identifying how you can give back to others.

As a reminder, in our last session, we worked on the goal of accepting that fear and pain are inescapable components of life. It's a fact that we all encounter moments of pain; however, these moments don't have to shape your identity. In addition to disentangling yourself from your fears and pain, it's time to shift your focus toward embracing the concept of your Best Possible Self and actively working toward embodying that ideal. At the end of the day, we all seek a sense of self-worth and the belief that we're living up to our inherent potential. Part of what contributes to a profound sense of confidence and overall well-being is our ability to connect with others meaningfully and offer something back to the world. Bearing this in mind, our ultimate goal today goes beyond personal growth; it's about finding ways to harness our passions, skills, and expertise to give back and leave a positive impact on the world.

CBT intervention: Your Declaration of Independence
Why a Declaration of Independence?

Before our next, and final, CBT exercise, we must have a short history lesson, because as we all know, if we do not know where we have come from, we will continue to make the same mistakes. So bear with me; I promise this will all make sense in a minute.

The United States' *Declaration of Independence*, written in 1776 by Thomas Jefferson, declared the United States' freedom from British rule. It states that everyone has basic rights like life, liberty, and the pursuit of happiness. Governments should get their power from the people and must protect these rights.

While there are many aspects of the 1776 US Declaration of Independence that should rightly be viewed critically in the modern day, particularly with a view to equality, we are going to take what is useful from it to use here as a metaphor, the message being: "We choose to govern our own selves and determine our own destiny."

And yes, you probably guessed it: You are going to compose your own personal Declaration of Independence. We will follow the format of four distinct sections: *Preamble, Indictment of Grievances, Denunciation and Justification,* and *Conclusions and Rights.* Use the page with the fancy scroll to write the introduction to your Declaration of Independence. Let's take it one section at a time.

Introduction and preamble

The introduction explains the reasons why the colonies wanted to break free from British rule. The US Declaration of Independence starts with:

> When in the course of human events, it becomes necessary for one people to dissolve the political bands which have connected them with another, and to assume among the powers of the earth, the separate and equal station to which the Laws of Nature and of Nature's God entitle them, a decent respect to the opinions of mankind requires that they should declare the causes which impel them to the separation.

Write your Declaration of Independence, liberating yourself from the constraints imposed by the thoughts and behaviors that hinder your progress in life. This statement signifies your desire to break free from these oppressive influences.

Start by writing "When in the course of human events, it becomes necessary for me to dissolve my connection with (fear, anger, substances, insecurity...whatever it is you have been working on for this whole book)..."

Take a moment to express how you have felt oppressed and controlled and state that you do not want to continue living that way. Elaborate as much as you want or keep it short and precise. This is your Declaration of Independence.

My client Erin's story revolved around post-college uncertainty, where she grappled with the direction of her life despite passion for her role as a fitness coach. Filled with apprehension and a sense of being adrift, Erin's Declaration of Independence began with these words:

> When in the course of human events, it becomes necessary for me to dissolve my connection with the fear of the unknown, uncertainty and discomfort and negative thoughts...

Indictment

This section provides a record of the instances where the king (allegedly) consistently violated the rights and liberties of the Americans, demonstrating a pattern of harm.

Here, you are going to state all the ways that your negative thoughts and fears have controlled you and caused you harm. What did your negative thoughts and fears make you do? What did they keep you from doing? You can write this as a list or in paragraph form.

> For Erin this next section was pretty short and straight to the point. She wrote:

> My fears of the unknown controlled me by not allowing me to get to my goals, fulfil my dreams, get to my dreams, or feel free. My fear of the unknown made me avoid making important decisions.

Denunciation

The section is crucial. It lists the wrongs suffered under British rule, explaining why revolution was necessary. By highlighting these alleged abuses and affirming basic human rights like life and liberty, it not only justifies independence but also sets the groundwork for the new nation's values.

This is where you get to proudly state everything that you will put in place to live a healthier life. These are the behaviors, thoughts and responses that will bring you that long-term sense of happiness and calm that you seek. In other words, these are your rules that you create to protect your freedoms. This is where you can really maintain life-long emotional wellness.

Ask yourself:

- What guidelines and routines will cultivate a life free from those detrimental thoughts that led me to this book?

- What are the healthy daily or weekly habits that will safe-guard you against reverting to self-destructive patterns? Examples include:

  - Setting a healthy bedtime routine.

  - Making healthy eating choices.

  - Surrounding yourself with positive and supportive people.

In this section, Erin made a pivotal decision to alter her behaviors, a choice that would ultimately free her from the grip of uncertainty and regain control over her life. She wrote:

I will set up these rules of behaviors and eventually they will become habits that I will live by.

- I will get 7–8 hours of sleep most nights.

- I will journal or meditate in the mornings, as a way to set the tone of my day to come.

- I will not beat myself up when I am not perfect. In fact, I will implement the 80/20 rule where I will make healthy choices 80% of the time and be gentle on myself the other 20% of the time.

- I will practice yoga at least once a week.

- I will continue to teach others.

- I will be open to learning from others.

- I will eat slowly and mindfully while sitting down.
- I will breathe.

Conclusion and rights

This section reiterates the inherent and unalienable rights of all individuals, such as life, liberty, and the pursuit of happiness.

Finally, you get to declare the freedoms that you will gain once you embrace the healthier version of you. What rights will you have once you are no longer being controlled by negative thoughts and fear? Examples include:

- The right to happiness and contentment.

- The right to pursue higher education or a desired career.

- The right to positive and supportive relationships.

- The right to choosing responses that will positively enhance relationships.

- The right to the feelings of balance and emotional wellness.

Erin concluded her Declaration of Independence with:

I now have the freedom to pursue happiness, contentment, fulfillment, and positivity. I have the right to healthy and supportive relationships. I have the right to travel and adventure. I have the right to NO restrictions.

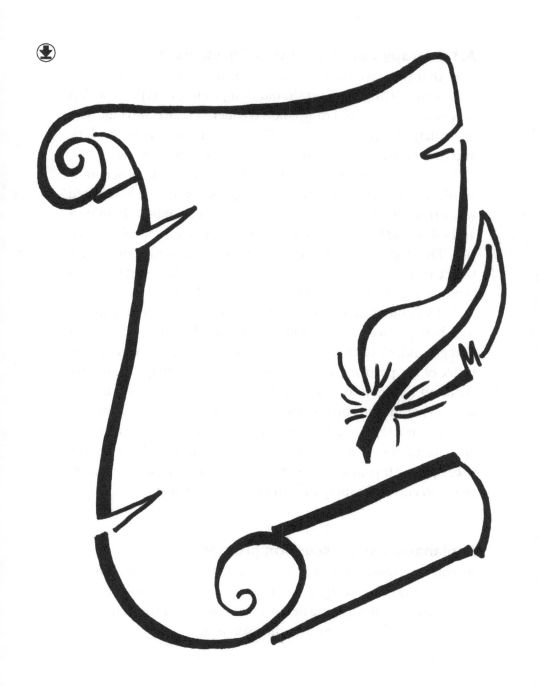

Art Therapy exercise: State of Wellness flag

Now that you have written your Declaration of Independence, it only seems fitting that you should design a flag to represent that new state of wellness. Using colored paper, scissors, and glue, you will collage together your flag. Think about what shapes, colors, and numbers will represent your new state of well-being.

For example, the colors of the US flag were not chosen arbitrarily. In 1777, the Continental Congress meticulously selected white to symbolize purity and innocence, red to embody hardiness and valor, and blue to represent vigilance, perseverance, and justice. The flag's shapes and numbers also hold significance, with the 13 stripes representing the original 13 colonies and the stars symbolizing the constituent states (currently 50).

Select colors that resonate deeply with your inner sense of well-being. Once you've found these colors, designate one as your background. Next, choose shapes or symbols that are the representative of the person you're evolving into. These shapes may have surfaced in previous drawings throughout this transformative journey, or maybe you will pick ones that are completely new to you. When integrating multiple shapes into your design, take into account the meaning behind the specific number of shapes you use. Approach your design with the same level of intentionality that you currently apply to your choices and behaviors.

Explanation and discussion prompts

As you have done with each previous exercise, take some time to reflect on the following questions. These prompts will serve as valuable tools for engaging in reflective journal writing, reminding you to delve even deeper into the exercises.

1. How did it feel while you were creating this flag?

2. Describe your flag—the colors, the shapes, numbers.

3. What meaning can be read into this flag?

4. What would you call your new state?

Additional exercises, follow up, and next steps: What you are carrying/holding (4th time)

One last drawing if you're up for it! Let's return to some of your drawings earlier in this process. Add something you can give/ share with others.

> As you may recall, Erin concluded her Declaration of Independence by declaring her freedom to pursue happiness, the right to healthy relationships, and the unrestricted ability to travel and adventure. She created her flag as a representation of these ideas. To convey this, she opted for striking neon colors: fluorescent green, bright yellow, electric pink, and vivid orange. Erin explained that she loves colors and the concept of brightness and light.
>
> Erin's flag had a theme of nature, with shapes that symbolized mountains, trees, and the ocean, which had repeatedly surfaced in her previous drawings.
>
> What adds an intriguing dimension to her creative process is her unconscious repurposing of a zig-zag or lightning bolt shape. In earlier sessions of the Creative Cognitive Therapy Method, Erin's drawings occasionally featured this lightning bolt shape, which symbolized negative energy, chaos, and confusion. Remarkably, Erin unconsciously repositioned this very lightning bolt by simply turning it on its side, effectively transforming it into a representation of mountains. What's even more astonishing is that Erin didn't initially realize it was the same shape until I pointed it out during our discussion.

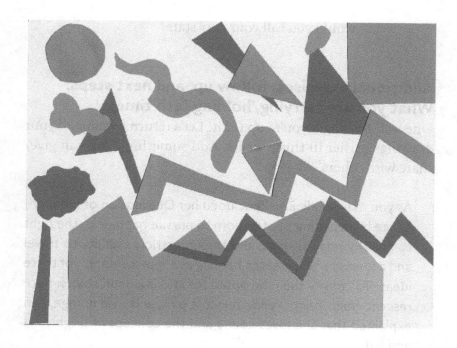

Art Therapy's unique ability to tap into the subconscious mind enables artworks to unveil connections and insights that might remain hidden during conventional conversations. This underscores the essential role of the discussion prompts within the Art Therapy process. These prompts provided Erin with a valuable opportunity to articulate the symbolism within her artwork. Erin candidly shared her deep affection for mountains, and, in a profound twist of interpretation, she also viewed them as a metaphor for converting uncertainty and chaos into inner strength.

What if, right now, you decided to embrace Brené Brown's powerful notion that "Love and belonging is a birthright and NOT something you have to earn"? Picture for a moment how it would feel to carry that belief with you. Imagine the freedom and strength it would bring, knowing that you are inherently deserving of love and belonging.

You've made remarkable progress throughout your journey with the Creative Cognitive Therapy Method, and it's truly commendable! I want to express my genuine pride in your achievements thus far. I'm filled with excitement for your path that lies ahead. It's essential to recognize that what you've accomplished is the foundation, a solid base upon which you can continue to build. To sustain the newfound freedoms and well-being you've attained, it's crucial to integrate these healthy behaviors into your daily life consistently. The final chapter will delve into the topic of maintenance, providing you with valuable insights and strategies to ensure the enduring benefits of your journey.

News of Erin: A few months after she and I worked together, Erin made a fearless decision to move to Austin, TX, where she is happy, healthy, and thriving.

NOTES FOR THERAPISTS

Alright, by now you know the drill... Start this session by introducing the quotation and discussing our goals. Next, have your client read their "Best Possible Self" statement out loud, and engage in a meaningful discussion as needed. Afterward, dedicate some time to revisit the progress made during the past nine sessions together. Check in with your client: How are they doing? What changes or shifts have they noticed? What areas require more attention, and what are they prepared to let go of?

Now, guide your client through the "Declaration of Independence" exercise. Ensure they have ample time to write it out, either in their notebook or on the fun scroll provided in this workbook.

As we approach the end of this tenth session, encourage your client to create their personal "State of Wellness Flag" as their final Art Therapy intervention with you. Have them share their experience of creating the collage and the symbolism behind the colors and images in their flag.

For the concluding homework assignment, suggest that

your client revisits the "What you are carrying/holding" drawing. This time, have them incorporate an element of sharing something with others.

In the event that this is your final session with them, consider assigning this homework as a means for them to independently continue their self-care journey. However, if your clients wish to continue therapy, I recommend a short break, perhaps a few weeks or a month, to allow them to integrate their newfound behaviors, thoughts, and self-care practices into their daily routine. You can then reconvene for maintenance as needed.

CHAPTER ELEVEN

Summary and Next Steps

Congratulations! You've successfully completed the entire Creative Cognitive Therapy Method, and that's no small feat. It may not have been an easy journey, demanding both your time and a willingness to step out of your comfort zone. But you've persevered, and for that, you should be proud.

Yet, this isn't the end; rather, it marks the beginning of a new chapter. The insights and tools you've gained are the foundation upon which you'll continue to build a happier, healthier, and more fulfilled life. Your path forward is filled with endless possibilities, and I'm excited about the positive transformations that await you.

Let me share a personal story to illustrate what is to come after this book. When I was 39 years old, I made a decision that would change not only my life but also how I understood the concept of character. I enrolled my eight-year-old daughter in a martial arts program. As I sat in the dojo week after week, watching my daughter in her lessons, I found myself intrigued. I decided to enroll myself in the adult mixed martial arts (MMA) classes they offered. I started as a white belt, and it was a great workout. Within four months, I had progressed to a yellow belt, and felt a remarkable increase in my physical strength and stamina. I formed friendships with fellow students, and my visits to the dojo became a four-times-a-week routine. With determination and dedication, I continued my journey and proudly earned my green belt. Then, after a year of training, I advanced to the blue belt. MMA wasn't just a workout; it had become an integral part of my identity.

After four years of donning my *gi* and showing up at the dojo five times a week, I reached the pinnacle—the black belt. It was a monumental achievement (I even broke a brick with my bare hand), one that filled me with pride and humility. However, my sensei, Mr. Josh, delivered a perspective-altering message. He explained that earning the black belt wasn't the culmination of my training; it was merely the beginning. He used a metaphor that struck a chord with me—kindergarten. Before we can even start kindergarten, he said, we spend at least five years grasping the fundamentals like numbers and counting. Only then are we truly prepared to move onto concepts like addition, subtraction, and, eventually, complex algebra.

The message was clear: I had defined my goals, identified my sacrifices, and committed to change. By doing one thing consistently several times a week I'd gained strength, built a community, and cultivated confidence. But just like the foundation of learning, the real work had just begun.

Remember, your character isn't fixed or predetermined but is rather a result of your choices and actions over time. Cultivating positive habits and values serves to develop a strong and virtuous character. My martial arts journey had not only made me physically stronger but had also instilled in me the discipline, dedication, and the resilience required to build and maintain character.

As I share this story with you, remember that you too have set your goals, made sacrifices, and determined what you're willing to do differently. Now, you have a lifetime ahead of you to shape your character by implementing and maintaining healthy habits. Your journey is a marathon, not a sprint, and it's in the persistence of your efforts that you'll truly discover the depth of who you are.

Plutarch said it concisely, "Character is simply habit long continued,"[18] suggesting that who someone is at their core is primarily shaped by the habits they've cultivated and maintained over an extended period of time. Our actions and behaviors, when repeated consistently, become ingrained as habits, and these habits ultimately define our character.

I send you off....

Endnotes

1   Hoffman, S. G., Smits, J. A., & Smith, B. N. (2020). "CBT for anxiety and depression: Advantages, limitations, and future directions." *Behaviour Research and Therapy, 128*, 103612.

2   Kaimal, G., Ray, K., & Muniz, J. (2016). "Reduction of Cortisol Levels and Participants' Responses Following Art Making." *Art Therapy: Journal of the American Art Therapy Association, 33*(2), 74–80.

3   https://online.yu.edu/wurzweiler/blog/prochaska-and-diclementes-stages-of-change-model-for-social-workers

4   www.goodreads.com/quotes/551027-yesterday-i-was-clever-so-i-wanted-to-change-the

5   https://madaboutmybody.com/2019/09/11/your-body-hears-everything-your-mind-says

6   www.counseling.org/news/aca-blogs/aca-counseling-corner/aca-member-blogs/2015/03/23/art-therapy-anxiety-is-it-just-child-s-play

7   Weekes, C. (2020). *Hope and Help for Your Nerves: End Anxiety Now*. New York: Penguin, 42–43.

8   Weekes, C. (2020). *Hope and Help for Your Nerves: End Anxiety Now*. New York: Penguin, 42–43.

9   Tolle, E. (2004). *The Power of Now: A Guide to Spiritual Enlightenment.* Novato, CA: New World Library.

10 Mueller, P. A., & Oppenheimer, D. M. (2014). The pen is mightier than the keyboard: Advantages of longhand over laptop note taking. *Psychological Science, 25*, 1159–1168.

11 Laozi, and Mitchell, S. (2006). *Tiao Te Ching: A New English Version*. New York: HarperPerennial.

12 https://daniellepa.com/how-have-you-changed-celebrating-evolution

13 https://youtu.be/fnzOKo5Vr2A?si=SAO187caTB3FeBP2

14 Meevissen, Y. M. C., Peters, M. L., & Alberts, H. J. E. M. (2011). "Become more optimistic by imagining a Best Possible Self: Effects of a two-week intervention." *Journal of Behavior Therapy and Experimental Psychiatry, 42*(3), 371–378.

15 Meevissen, Y. M. C., Peters, M. L., & Alberts, H. J. E. M. (2011). "Become more optimistic by imagining a Best Possible Self: Effects of a two-week intervention." *Journal of Behavior Therapy and Experimental Psychiatry, 42*(3), 371–378.

16 Brown, B. & Hai, R. (2012). "Being vulnerable about vulnerability: Q&A with Brené Brown", *TEDBlog*, 16 March. Available at: https://blog.ted.com/being-vulnerable-about-vulnerability-qa-with-brene-brown/comment-page-2

17   Brown, B. (2010). *The Gifts of Imperfection: Let Go of Who You Think You Are Supposed to Be and Embrace Who You Are.* Minneapolis, MN: Hazelden.
18   www.brainyquote.com/authors/plutarch-quotes